"WELLNESS":
A NEW WORD FOR ANCIENT IDEAS

"WELLNESS":
A NEW WORD FOR ANCIENT IDEAS

A Study on Ancient Chinese, Egyptian,
Greek, Indian, And Iranian Medicine

Iris Efthymiou - Egleton

Copyright © 2017 by Iris Efthymiou - Egleton.

ISBN: Softcover   978-1-5434-8730-5
           eBook   978-1-5434-8729-9

All rights reserved. No part of this book may be reproduced or transmitted in any form or by any means, electronic or mechanical, including photocopying, recording, or by any information storage and retrieval system, without permission in writing from the copyright owner.

Any people depicted in stock imagery provided by Thinkstock are models, and such images are being used for illustrative purposes only. Certain stock imagery © Thinkstock.

Print information available on the last page.

Rev. date: 09/18/2017

To order additional copies of this book, contact:
Xlibris
800-056-3182
www.Xlibrispublishing.co.uk
Orders@Xlibrispublishing.co.uk
731458

CONTENTS

Disclaimer ix
Author's Note xi
Prologue xv
Introduction xxiii

Whatever Happened to Good Old Ms. Wellness? 1
    You Want Information? Well, We Got Plenty! (Strike #1) 5
    Or Do You Want Similarities? Well, We Got Plenty Too!
    (Strike #2) 6
    Plenty of Forgotten Wisdom, As Well! (Strike #3) 8

First Part of the Journey: The Asian Tour 10

Balance: The One to Open Our Eyes is CHINA! 14
    The History of Traditional Chinese Medicine 14
    The Golden Chamber of Chang Chung-Ching 18
    The Prolific Sun Simiao 19
    Daoism: Yet Another Influential Factor on Medicine 22
    Treatment Methods 23
    The Humble Confucius 25
    The Five Elements Theory 25
    Our Beloved Acupuncture 27
    Herbal Medicine 30
    Have You Heard of Moxibustion? 32
    Massage: A Great Way to Rest from the Rat Race 33
    Getting Enlightened with the Fine Art of Qi Gong 33
    Tai Chi: You Have Heard It; Do You Really Know It? 36
    Diet 37

- Yin and Yang: A Can't-Be-With-You-Can't-Live-Without-You Story 38
- Dualities in the Yin-Yang Theory 39
- TCM Does Not Come Without Its Strengths and Particularities 41

The Master of Herbal Compounds, aka India 48
- The History of Ancient Indian Medicine 48
- The Innovative Charaka and His Balance Theory 49
- Nip/Tuck 50
- Reaching the Core with Ayurveda 52
- Herbal Medicine 56
- Looking for an Excuse to Have a Drink? 59
- Oils to the Rescue! 60
- Yoga and Meditation: Two of Celebrities' Most-loved Practices 61
- Other Medical Systems 63

Healing with Ample Professionality in Iran 65
- The History of Persian (Ancient Iranian) Medicine: A Brief Presentation 65
- Medical Practitioner Types 67
- Avesta 68
- Let's Meet the Most Emblematic Personalities 71
- Nipping & Tucking in Ancient Iran 76
- The Four Humors 77
- The Resourceful Rhazes 79
- Remarkable Writings 82
- Herbal Medicine 83
- The Yasht Classification of Physicians 85
- Exceptional Facts 85

Second Part of the Journey: A Mediterranean Cruise 88

Treating with a Pinch of Artistry in Egypt 93
   A Short History of Ancient Egyptian Medicine 93
   Suffering from Frequent Diseases 96
   Surgery and Circumcision 98
   The Significance of Well-Reserved Papyri 101
   Diet and Dental Health 101
   Herbal Wellness 104
   Exceptional Facts 105
   The Classification of Physicians 107
   Magic VS. Logic 109
   Hygiene 111

Curing Warrior Wounds in Greece 113
   Disease Meant Divine Punishment: A Karmic View! 113
   The History of Ancient Greek Medicine:
   A Brief Presentation 115
   Surgery and Surgical Instruments 117
   The 4 Elements & The 4 Humors:
   How interconnected are they? 120
   The Confluence Between Diet and Health:
   They Do Meet Somewhere! 124
   How Were the Medical Professions Perceived? 125
   Hippocrates – Part I 127
   What Is Naturopathy? 133
   The Always Present Herbal Medicine 135
   Move Your Body 138
   The Father of Medicine – Part II 138
   Let's Go Meet a Few More Notable Personalities
   (and Their Contribution to Medicine) 142
   Hypnosis 145
   Melampus, the First Psychiatrist 149
   Mental Health Issues 150

Epilogue	153
Appendix 1	167
Appendix 2	169
Appendix 3	171
Sources	173
Books	177

DISCLAIMER

The research for this book was a mixture of paper and online sources relating to the history of medicine. The medical information provided (medical information relating to disease, injury, drugs, herbs and other treatments, medical tools and devices) is of a general nature and has a historical point of view. It should not be construed as an attempt to render a medical opinion or otherwise engage in the practice of medicine. And this was not my aim when putting all that information together; this book is not intended as a substitute for the medical advice of physicians. The reader should consult a physician in matters relating to their health and particularly with respect to any symptoms that may require diagnosis or medical attention.

AUTHOR'S NOTE

I decided to write this book not long after my first book "Trends in Health Care: A Global Challenge" was released. That first book was focused on the future of the medical field, so this time around I had to travel back in time. Winston Churchill has said 'The farther back you can look, the farther forward you are likely to see.' Of course, many others have been quoted with saying something similar like 'to move forward, you must look back', but I prefer the Churchill version that incorporates a capability and a chance to prolong one's limits instead of almost dictating an obligation. People who meet me soon notice that I am both traditional and evolutionary. And one's personality reflects in their books, even if they are not of literary nature. So, in my contrasting case, it shows in my will to both study the past and project to the future. I always believed that the past is not something to leave behind untouched. In a way, it stays alive and current, therefore it should be respected and study of the past should be viewed as a useful tool for building a better, more stable and more desirable future.

Fortunately, in this journey back in time, I was not alone. I had the strong encouragement of my husband and the wholehearted support of my entire family throughout the studying and gathering information and putting the puzzle pieces of the past together and finally shaping it all into another book in my humble collection. I also had an amazing copilot, my text editor, Konstantinos Kotidis, who affectionately, almost paternally, oversaw this project from conception to fruition. He made suggestions, corrected all my grammatical errors without lecturing, and we had such a wonderful collaboration.

The study of history is inevitably a conversation with the present; the study of medical history is inevitably a conversation with contemporary medicine. Studying the history of medicine, one can learn about the constraints and prospects of the human condition across time and cultures.

The Swiss medical historian Henry E. Sigerist has pointed out that "there is no such thing as a definite history, because interpretation and evaluation change over time." I believe that, in their 'Companion Encyclopedia of the History of Medicine,' Bynum and Porter kind of complete Sigerist's idea when they say that "the two most important tasks for medical historians are now to concentrate on comparative and on synthetic studies across cultural, national, and social lines."

PROLOGUE

Medicine is definitely one of the most crucial — if not *the* most crucial — necessities for all people. A broad historical knowledge and perspective could help us understand the nature of medicine within our society. Obviously, its importance has been there since the ancient times. It is derived from the Latin words *ars medicina* which mean "the art of healing." It is of course a branch of the health sciences that is concerned with maintaining or restoring human health through the study, diagnosis, treatment and also possible prevention of disease, injury and other damage to a human body, mind or soul.

And let's not forget — though it might be extremely painful to accept it, and for us women even more — that once we get older, some kind of medication will become an indispensable part of our life. I mean, even the luckiest, the most fortunate health-wise person in the world will grow old and suffer from a chronic condition. Among the most common health concerns for seniors are arthritis, heart disease, respiratory diseases, Alzheimer's Disease, osteoporosis, diabetes, pneumonia, and oral health.

Another necessity that we used to forget is wellbeing. And I said "used to" because little by little wellbeing and its little sister, wellness, are increasingly integrated in our lives. They are entering the minds and consciousnesses of more and more countries and peoples. First, let's see the relation and the differences between those two siblings. Wellbeing refers to our mental, emotional and spiritual state, which is of course impacted by our physical health. On the other hand, wellness relates primarily to our physical state, which in turn is very much affected by our emotional state and goes hand in hand with our spiritual state and mood. So, while those two are closely related, they are different.

It's pretty clear that we need both wellness and wellbeing in order to thrive. Sometimes, it seems like wellness is just a part of wellbeing, but in reality, that's incorrect, because wellness includes not just an individual's physical health, but also the required state of mind. It is a mistake to think that physical health means having a well-shaped body; what it really incorporates is keeping our body properly and wisely fed, cleaned and trained — not focusing on the appearance part but on the health part. And one last note I would like to make around their definitions is that nowadays we have shaped many types of wellbeing, such as social, emotional, psychological, physical and economic wellbeing.

In any case, what's more significant is that feeling good inside and out, thinking positively about life and everything around it, as well as taking equal care of our body and soul are all of utmost importance. Now, if I'm to add a personal comment, as I love to do always, I'd say that even though the two terms are not interchangeable technically, they do become interchangeable if we approach them from a mental point of view, since they both incorporate the notions of internal as well as external balances. It's just that they focus on two different elements of it all. Everybody goes through different periods, at least health-wise, in their lifetime; ones where there were few or no problems at all, where everything seem to flow as easily as humanly possible and ones where various problems (related to health, work, family, friends, finances, or a combination of those) seem to never end. **Each time we find ourselves in a moment of bliss and prosperity, we tend to take it as a given** more and more, but the truth is that life is much associated with problems, worries, and issues and, thus, we have to be strong, willing and able to deal with them and solve them — once and for all, if possible.

Humans have long sought advice from those with knowledge or skill in healing. Paleopathology and other historical records allow an examination of how ancient societies dealt with illness and outbreak. Instinctively, all people want to face any ordeal ASAP and various sciences, tools, tricks, methods and techniques were developed towards that goal: agriculture, weapons, the arts, and of course medicine. Stopping the spread of infectious disease was always of utmost importance for maintaining a healthy society.

In this day and age, people have greater and greater demands concerning their health condition and overall wellbeing and doctors respond the same way. Not being sick is not the desired goal anymore; now, it is having the best health condition, being as fit as it gets, or being "rich and thin," as a very common expression goes. Obviously, we are talking about the Western world, that is the European and American continents, because if we see this more globally, we will find out that the notion of health widely varies in different cultures and nations.

In general, all those different definitions do have some common ground; for instance, they all have a state of harmony at their core. We can see that the necessary state of mind accompanying a person's wellness was discovered early on. It can also be seen as a continuous struggle, as part of a dialectical process, as an internal balance of the human body, as a set of abilities, as the result of a conscious responsible conduct, and the list goes on. For the Greek philosopher Diogenes, the key to a healthy life and conduct was asceticism; for the Stoics, the healthiest state of the soul was a kind of sangfroid (apathy); for Epicurus, it was the serenity of the mind (ataraxy). Marcus Aurelius sought the calmness of the mind (*tranquilitas animi*) through self-control; the Persian physician and philosopher Avicenna asserted that the soul can only be cured through empathy and understanding; in the early Christian years, the *Christus medicus* movement saw health as the vicinity to God and so, people tried to achieve good health by embracing and imitating the life of Jesus Christ.

As a human being, I find it particularly satisfying and fulfilling that there is at least one scientific field where all humanity is united in the name of its progress. Indeed, no matter where a medical scientist may come from, no matter their color, religion, height, social class, age, mother tongue, political beliefs, their contribution is immediately globally respected and recognized to an unprecedentedly high degree; it is almost enviable. The only thing in which the entire medical community is interested is the new discovery, the new step, the new piece of information or the new cure. The scientists of Islam, for instance, got many ideas from Greece and India, they combined and evolved them. And now, modern medicine owes a lot to the work of Islam's doctors. This kind of practice showed for the first time that science surpasses political borders and religious relations as it is a body of knowledge that benefits all people.

In this book, it will become clear that medical practitioners and medical scientists of any kind, field and subfield respected and valued the work of their predecessors. It is admirable that humanity has been incessantly honoring the undeniable priority that is healthcare. It happened since the very beginning, since the earliest antiquity. In a world where social, political, moral and/or financial issues and crises seem to be an unavoidable constant, medicine stands alone as the field that is in a constant state of progress – a field that always moves forward.

This can be verified by watching the evening news as well. There are wars, terrorism, financial crises, major political incompetence, and moral ambiguities of every kind you could possibly imagine. However, when it comes to medicine, it is always about some new, miraculous cure that may lead to new theories and new discoveries, about another conjoined twins' separation surgery that was successful against the odds, about a new medical institution etc. Just like everyone else, I am not just a human being brought here by a stork. I am a daughter, a wife, a sister, even more importantly a mother, and I need that hope; I need those pieces of good news. And if the medical field sometimes moves backwards, it is to find answers, and in general more information, in the past. Because, as we will see, the medical knowledge of the past, Traditional Medicine practices, and numerous ancient concepts are still relevant today.

Unfortunately, untreatable diseases such as cancer, AIDS, and multiple sclerosis still exist, but so does hope. And so do scientific research and experiments. While doing research for this book, an insane amount of information that was really hard to grasp came to my attention and most of it made me appreciate like never before the fact that I get to live in this day and age when most diseases are dealt with by swallowing a single pill or getting one single vaccine, usually as a kid or even a baby. Even though ancient civilizations, such as the ones we are going to study, had pretty much laid the grounds for all future generations, I am sure they would be astounded to see the medical advances of our era.

By the way, I would not want to hide my pride as a Greek to find out to what degree exactly my motherland and my ancestors form an integral part in the history and evolution of medicine and medical practice. Ancient Greeks travelled to other countries to collect information and they equally offered their own developed knowledge and new useful discoveries to other civilizations and to newer generations. They were also the first ones to develop a specialized medical vocabulary covering several medical fields, such as internal and external anatomy, cardiology, dentistry, obstetrics, disease nomenclature and many more.

Generally, ancient medical systems stressed the importance of reducing illness through divination and ritual. Other codes of behavior and dietary protocols were also widespread in the ancient world. During the Zhou Dynasty in China, doctors suggested exercise, meditation and temperance to preserve one's health. The Chinese closely link health with spiritual well-being. Health regimes in ancient India focused on oral health as the best method for a healthy life. The Talmudic code created rules for health which stressed ritual cleanliness, connected disease with certain animals and created diets. Other examples include the Mosaic Code and Roman baths and aqueducts.

Mirko Grmek has written a very interesting book on diseases, a work that defies their easy classification. In it, he adopts the environmental approach to explaining how a disease is spread. He supports that, in general, diseases occur when two causal factors, one genetic and one external, intersect. His main conclusion, which is very interestingly implicit, can be summed up in that most diseases appear due to a conjunction of an innate weakness and a vast multitude of environmental factors.

Every generation rewrites history, not so much because it can be done in a better way, but mainly because the questions and the aspects of interest change with time. The questions about the role and nature of medicine change not only with time but also differ within the cultures of the world. The medical profession and the moral limits that may accompany it are no longer at the center of attention; now, we are focused at the social meaning of disease, at a holistic approach of the patient's life and world. The historical study has shifted in the same way: the new emphasis is the social history and not the politico-economical history anymore. Studying the history of population change, women, sexuality, and family encouraged the examination of historical patterns of disease and, even more so, epidemic disease. The latter caused changes in the organization of cultural norms and values, institutions and intellect; changes that are worthy of being extensively studied.

As anyone can easily imagine, the history of medicine is pretty long and equally remarkable. Since the dawn of humanity, there had to be a way to alleviate, to cure the sick from all kinds of ailment or disease. When we talk about ancient medicine in particular, there are at least five countries that come to mind; alphabetically, these are China, Egypt, Greece, India and Iran. This means that, in this study, we are going to travel not only back in time but also to three different continents. So, we start off this journey by meeting China, India and Iran in the first chapter, and then, Egypt and Greece in the second one.

The main conclusion when studying the history and achievements of ancient medicine is that it remains key for every new discovery. It may be dated, but it is not outdated. It still is and should remain the basis for every direction that modern-day health sciences choose. From the benefits of countless herbs to the influence of psychology on our physical health, our ancestors have laid admirable foundations for us to utilize. As for the content that is studied and presented for each of these ancient countries, the elements that are analyzed are:

- the history of each country's traditional medicine's birth, formation, gradual development and progress,
- the philosophy around what is disease, why it exists, and why people have to suffer because of it,
- the various types of treatment and medical approaches,
- the sector of herbal medicine, with a special mention of enough herbs and medicinal plants and their use,
- the influence received by and/or given to other cultures,
- the most renowned and prolific personalities in the history of medicine along with their esteemed works,
- and, finally, any other information that is brilliant and noteworthy and that would be considered an omission if not included.

INTRODUCTION

In principle, modern-day medicine is a unique and united entity all around the world, even though we can find many varying mentalities around it. I already mentioned how medical scientists of all nationalities are working together and communicating each and every new discovery – in full detail – with each other. In ancient times, the various traditional medicines of different countries may have had several similarities (which is somewhat unavoidable, since we are talking about pretty much the same diseases), but they also had fundamental philosophical and mental differences. Each culture had its very own approach to the subject, its very own beliefs and POVs.

Considering the fact that technology was absent – unborn, one might say, – communication was determinately limited. As a result, once having traveled and imparted the new information, there remained the difficulty of comprehending and then transferring the fundamental cultural elements that were found in the core of said information. So, basically, once the healthcare professionals of country A have grasped the basics of the medical remedies and treatments of country B (that is, of a whole different culture), the greatest challenge is still ahead. And that is understanding the beliefs and attitudes about sickness that drove the foreign medico-philosophical approach and practice.

On the one hand, Western medicine tends to approach diseases by assuming that they are due to an external force, such as a virus or bacteria, or a slow degeneration of the functional ability of the body. Disease is either physical or mental.

On the other hand, the Eastern approach perceives the body as a whole, and theorizes that all parts of it are intimately interconnected. Each organ has a mental as well as a physical function. We could argue that the Eastern approach integrated the philosophies of wellness and wellbeing from earlier on and more consciously too. Perhaps a melding of the two belief systems would be ideal, but it isn't easy in hectic settings or crisis situations to bring such divergent belief systems together during medical care and consultation.

The observation-based prediction of an illness' development was an important step in the history of medicine, as it allowed physicians to identify specific illnesses that responded to individualized, and therefore better and more effective, treatment. There were shamans, there were pagan priests, and then there was Hippocrates. Every doctor that has walked on this earth knows about him, since they had to take the Hippocratic oath – after having studied him thoroughly, of course. Shamans and pagan priests used various rituals and medical techniques to cure ailments. Through these rituals and their "magic," they sometimes arrived at a cure (many times by luck, as one might expect) that passed on from generation to generation into oral tradition and memory. Herbs, acupuncture and, yes, even prayer were commonly used to cure or alleviate those in need.

With the advent of medical sciences, we have started living a better and longer life. There are certain things in life that are out of our control; for instance, an unexpected accident, an unwished disease or an unwanted failure of any of our body organs. These are some of the cases when we consciously understand the importance of medicine. **Given that all the cells in our body carry the very same DNA, it is fascinating how our organs look so unlike and function so differently.** Thanks to our progress in epigenetics, we have learned that cells use their genetic material in different ways, and as genes are switched on and off, an astonishing level of differentiation occurs within our body. Epigenetics is the science that describes the cellular processes determining whether a certain gene will be transcribed and translated into its corresponding protein. The message can be conveyed through small and reversible chemical modifications to chromatin. Epigenetic modifications can occur in response to environmental stimuli, with diet being one of the most important ones. I know it was kind of expected, given the subject of the study, but since the mechanisms by which diet affects epigenetics are not yet fully understood, I will have to give a couple of clear examples to get the message across.

During the winter of 1944–1945, the Netherlands suffered a terrible famine as a result of the German occupation, and the population's nutritional intake dropped to fewer than 1000 calories per day. However, women continued to conceive and give birth during these hard times, and these children, who were exposed to calorie restrictions while in their mother's uterus, have a higher rate of chronic conditions such as diabetes, cardiovascular disease and obesity than their siblings, as revealed by recent studies. The first months of pregnancy seem to have had the greatest effect on disease risk. The exact epigenetic alterations may not be clear as of yet, but it was discovered that people who were exposed to famine in utero have a lower degree of methylation of a gene implicated in insulin metabolism than their siblings who were not exposed (Heijmans et al., 2008).

The effects of early diet on epigenetics are also clearly visible in honeybees – our second example. The difference between the sterile worker bees and the fertile queen has nothing to do with genetics; it is the diet that they followed when they were larvae. Larvae designated to become queens are fed exclusively with royal jelly, a substance secreted by worker bees, which switches on the gene program that results in the bee becoming fertile. As usual, there are examples with mice and rats too, but I chose not to bother you with those; let's talk humans instead! In humans, an insufficient uptake of folic acid is implicated in developmental conditions in humans, such as spina bifida and other neural tube defects. So, to prevent such problems, folic acid supplements are widely recommended for pregnant women.

Now, there are many food components that can cause epigenetic changes in our adult life. For example, broccoli and other vegetables can help increase histone acetylation. Soya, on the other hand, can help decrease DNA methylation in certain genes. Deficiencies in other essential molecules, such as Vitamin B12 and the mineral zinc, can too have effects on the levels of DNA methylation in our body, as revealed by studies in rodents and humans. And the list goes on with green tea, turmeric, and other foods. In general, epidemiological studies suggest that populations consuming large amounts of these foods appear to be less prone to certain diseases. Of course, a food may contain many different biologically active molecules and all foods undergo many transformations in our digestive system. Add to those two that every organism is different and you will get why it is so hard for the epigenetic modifications to be accurately measured. We already knew that diet plays a vital role in our health condition, right? In fact, people seem to have known that ever since ancient times, as we will find out. But who could imagine to what extent our dietary habits influence our health?

The scientific branch of medicine comprises all sorts of treatments that can be used to cure the human body. It also includes preventive systems that help us prevent many diseases. For example, there are numerous vaccinations nowadays for the prevention of diseases that were a true life-threatening menace in the (not as far as you might think) past. Two further examples are the aforementioned notions of wellness and wellbeing. A treatment, under the branch of medicine, is done through diet, drugs, exercise and other non-surgical means. Apart from curing some disease or healing a wound, medicine is also used to maintain good health at times. For instance, a diabetic individual must take medicine regularly to control the sugar level in their blood. Similarly, some people must take medicine daily in order to maintain the blood pressure of their body. So, medicine is also crucial for maintaining good health and not just restoring it.

There are many forms of medicine, such as allopathic, homeopathic and herbal. The latter is considered the best (healthiest and safest, in particular) in most cases, for the sole reason that it is made from natural ingredients only. Nature has always been a valuable source for medical products. Chinese, Ayurveda, Siddha, Unani, Tibetan... all medical systems make use of plants, simply because the latter can produce a diverse range of bioactive molecules. Obviously, herbal medicines have minimal toxicity, are cost-effective and pharmacologically active, providing an easy remedy for many ailments. All parts of a plant can be used to produce medicines. Herbal medicine makes use of berries, plant seeds, leaves, roots, peels, buds, stems, rhizomes, essential oils, barks and even flowers for medical purposes.

Although it used to be a form of medicine that was kept apart from the conventional medicine, today herbalism has reclaimed its well-deserved place in the mainstream medical practice worldwide and doctors recommend herbal medicines in many cases. Medicinal plants are considered an important source of new chemical substances with potential therapeutic effects that can be used to treat chronic and infectious diseases. Also, natural plant products can be the templates for new drug development. They have many interesting biological activities, such as gastroprotective, antidiabetic, antioxidant, antibacterial, anti-inflammatory, and antipyretic effects. The medicinal value of plants lies in the phytochemicals in them that produce a definite physiological action in the human body. Plants synthesize and accumulate in their cells a great variety of phytochemicals (such as tannins, flavonoids, phenolic compounds, glycosides, steroids, and saponins) that can control many human diseases.

Another thing that strikes me to the point where I cannot leave it uncommented is the good care that all physicians took of the findings of their predecessors. In fact, from antiquity to the early twentieth century, medical history has been dominated by a doxographic approach. Physicians have always been particularly eager to learn about the opinions of their predecessors and write them down in a more analytical and organized way. This has come to be a hallmark in the history of medicine. So, why is doxography no longer the way physicians choose to write down medical historiography? Possible explanations for this waning of interest include the increasing certainty and confidence afforded by the advances in science that have helped explain basic mechanisms of disease and therapy as well as the causal precision afforded by new methods that historians now use.

That same love and respect can be found in the Roman Empire, which came later and thus is (kind of) left out of this study. However,

I am going to implicitly give you the backstory, which can perfectly fill the "From Then On" part of this historical study. It is true that the Roman contribution to the history of medicine is often overlooked, with only Galen, of Greek origin, believed to be worth mentioning. Well, this is not the fairest thing for the Romans because they did put their excellent engineering skills to use in developing preventative medicine. They understood the role of dirt and poor hygiene in spreading disease and created aqueducts to ensure that the inhabitants of a city had access to clean water. Moreover, the Roman engineers installed elaborate sewage systems to carry the waste away. This is something that Europeans did not fully comprehend until the 19th century; before that period, sewage was still discharged close to drinking water.

The Romans may not have understood the exact mechanisms behind disease but their admirable level of personal hygiene and obsession with cleanliness certainly helped reduce the number of epidemics in the major cities. Furthermore, concerning surgery, they held the tradition of the Greeks. However, due to the fact that a Roman soldier was seen as a highly trained and valuable commodity, the military surgeons went on being developed into fine practitioners of their own art. Their refined procedures ensured that Roman soldiers had a much lower chance of dying from infection than those in the armies of their enemies.

When referring to the Roman influence on the history of medicine, Galen is the most illustrious name of it. This Greek physician, granted an expensive education by his merchant father, studied in the medical school of Pergamum and frequented the Asclepeions. In 161 AD., Galen moved to Rome, where he worked as a physician to the gladiators, which allowed him to study physiology and anatomy. Later in his life, he put his findings into writing and was the creator of many works on human physiology and the treatment of ailments. As his fame both as a physician and a lecturer spread, he went on to become the personal physician of three emperors: Marcus Aurelius, Commodus and Septimus Severus.

Much of the Hippocratic legacy was actually transmitted to the West through the writings of Galen, who dominated medical thinking for more than a millennium. Galen saw himself as extending and completing the framework of the Hippocratics. He wrote about all aspects of medicine. He codified the Hippocratic doctrine of the humors, but also consolidated an experimental dimension to medicine. Whereas the Hippocratics were content with careful observation, Galen went much further, offering anatomical and physiological accounts of what happened in health and disease.

When the Roman Empire split into the Western and Eastern Empires, the Western Empire, centered on Rome, fell into a massive decline and the art of medicine slowly lost the glory it once had, with the physicians becoming the flickering shadows of their esteemed predecessors and generally causing more harm than good. Western Europe would not appear again in the history of medicine until long after the decline of Islam.

In the Eastern Empire, based on Byzantium, physicians kept the knowledge and the skills passed from the Romans and the Greeks. This knowledge would form the basis of the Islamic medicine that would refine and improve medial techniques during the Islamic domination of the Mediterranean and Middle East. The history of Medicine would be written mostly in the Middle East and Asia for the next few centuries.

WHATEVER HAPPENED TO GOOD OLD MS. WELLNESS?

Wellness and wellbeing are concepts that have been forgotten, locked up in the drawers of dusty offices. They are not compatible with the modern lifestyle and the demanding goals we usually set. We use the terms, but do not apply their deep, true meaning. Much has been said already about the negative elements of the 21st-century lifestyle, like our lack of socializing, too much focusing on work and other profitable projects, disconnecting from mother nature, and sadly they are all true and not at all exaggerated.

This book is of medical interest and, in particular, of ancient medicine and its history. Medicine is a rapidly evolving scientific field that constantly cures previously incurable diseases. So, in a word, it can doubtlessly be described as miraculous. In recent years, I have read – I have had the blessing to read – numerous medical articles where scientists had well-founded hopes of curing cancer and HIV-infection once and for all. This point of view, the "curing" point of view, sounds very progressive and forward-looking and it is, but…

…on the other hand, this is the era when depression, anxiety and chronic stress are on the rise like never before in history. Which tells me that, when it comes to human health issues, the drawbacks of modern lifestyle largely outweigh its advantages, such as new drugs and new technologies. Hmm, really makes you think! And more precisely, it makes you think that we are doing many things – certainly not just one – wrong.

One of those many errors is believing that wellness is a synonym of good health or fitness. Well, wellness is not just the state of being... well! It is an integrated philosophy; it encompasses being fully aware of what living healthily means; it encompasses making mindful choices toward a lifestyle that is not only healthy but also serene, sustainable and fulfilling; it also encompasses wellbeing as a consciously chosen goal.

More than anything, the world we live in is characterized by interconnectedness. What we say, how we speak, what we do, how we act, even our feelings, moods, and emotions are directly affected by our life choices. The healthier we live, the healthier we feel. The stronger we feel, the stronger our decisions and initiatives are and the more upbeat we feel at work. It is all part of an ever-going circle.

Wellness refers to our wellbeing health-wise, family-wise, at work, at home, with our friends, psychologically, mentally and physically. No aspect of our life is excluded. I personally love the concept of wellness which incorporates living consciously and mindfully; living in a way that is healthy and also staying in the moment and enjoying life; living in the moment and, at the same time, taking care of ourselves in an ensuring way for the future. You see, this is the most realistic option if you want to lead an accomplished yet unanxious life. It's the combination that makes this concept brilliant. Bet you have all heard of theories like "live every day like it's your last day on Earth" or "save and prepare for the future." What such theories have in common is that they are too focused on one part of our life, leaving little room for the other, which renders them unpractical and unrealistic. We cannot turn back time, so we need both our present and future to be enjoyable.

Remember when I said how medicine is rapidly evolving a few paragraphs earlier? Well, this may be true, but the fact that some things remain the same is also true. No matter how many lab experiments are conducted and how many vaccines are invented, the way we live our life is a constant. What's happened is that modern-day pressure and tensions have taken away our tranquility and peace of mind. That, in turn, has led to people being unable to focus on what is truly important, to prioritize in a healthy way and to take care of themselves as they should. This has always happened and possibly always will, but it seems that currently we have reached a new high.

Thankfully, we already know the answer. It has been well-described as far back as two millennia ago. Before revealing anything, I would like to state how much I love it when medicine meets philosophy. So, Galen (129-210 AD), a prominent Greek physician and philosopher, has offered us many helpful writings about life and health. The part that probably interests me the most is the one concerning things — simple things — that everyone should do to have a better health status. The Roman-Empire-era physician has described the six necessary activities that can have but a beneficial effect on our health, whether we are sick or not. This following list can also serve as pieces of evidence that there are quite a few things that remain the same despite any progress or advancements. Note that the word 'activities' is used loosely; it might be a matter of actions, choices, or even thoughts. But, in any case, the usefulness of those six activities is beyond doubt.

First of all, breathing. Obviously, I'm not — well, technically, Galen wasn't, not me — talking about the mere act of inhaling and exhaling air to survive. In this particular case, breathing refers to deep, mindful breathing; and preferably, air that is clean and fresh! Also, it refers to breaths that we take to relax as much as we can; breaths to help us regain power; breaths to make us calm down and face whatever it is we have to face in our life, work etc. Decisions should be made with a clear mind. To be able to view an issue from multiple angles, you must be serene and calm. Otherwise, your brain will get stuck in one single point of view because of the dominating stress. So, deep breaths, everyone!

Second of all, eating (and drinking). That was probably an expected and easy one to guess. I see those regrets in your eyes, having wolfed down that family-size ice cream last night in front of the TV or having gobbled up one drink too many at the club. Alright now, I'm not going to lecture you on nutrition or make a list with fruit and vegetables in one column and sugar and pizzas in the other. At this point, my aim is for you to change the way you see food. Maybe you have heard the expression "you are what you eat." Don't worry, it is not meant to be taken literally; eating pork doesn't make you a pig. The expression refers to the close relation between your eating habits and your state of health. I know that food is one of the greatest joys of life and that 'eating what you please' sounds dreamy, but it is also chimerical, as all things that sound too good to be true. Anyway, the thing is that you should see the foods you eat as gifts to your body. Focus on a food's benefits instead of perceiving bad yet tasty foods as restrictions or limitations. That's the trick. After all, isn't it all a brain game?

Thirdly, exercise and rest. Our body is not made to stand still. It is made to act and then rest to regain forces and act again. Just like our mind, our body needs to be active and productive. Again, our perception of things plays a vital role. Exercise should not be seen as an activity of fatigue and exhaustion, but rather as a moment to take a break from the daily grind, a moment of uplift, a moment to take care of your body, helping your blood circulation come round, letting your muscles move and burning unneeded stored fat. And once your workout is done, make sure to take a breath; rushing back to work won't do.

Moving on to number four and there we find Sleep. Obviously, Galen did not refer to sleep in general. For example, catnaps, disco naps, and siestas are not included. We are supposed to sleep worry-free and not fitful, but our troubles seem to get in the way almost every night. Well, what Galen suggested is that we should reflect on the day we had and on the day that follows before going to bed, before even putting on our nightclothes. Any judgments, any decisions, any regrets, any criticism must not accompany us to the bed.

The fifth necessary activity has to do with our tranquility and state of mind. There were cases where Galen would diagnose a tumor or a dead fetus just by the patient's pulse and their agitation and disturbance. Having a clear state of mind expands to many things, such as taking care of yourself, of your obligations and duties, not procrastinating, not hiding behind false excuses and unreasonable justifications, facing any issue with bravery and in time, expressing your thoughts and feelings instead of repressing them, and getting a little further and more general, behaving with dignity and honesty.

"WELLNESS": A NEW WORD FOR ANCIENT IDEAS

Lastly, at number six, we find balance. Well, that is the actual goal. To find our balance. Balance is needed in everything. On one hand, it refers to our physiological balance, the one that our body needs in order to function properly and on the other hand, it refers to the balance of life. The balance of *our* life. In fact, it is our responsibility to find our balance point, the one that will help us stay sane and calm at all times and not lose our temper, even when things go very awry. This applies to virtually every single aspect of our life. For instance, when it comes to the way you dress, your balance point will encourage you to not dress too revealingly yet not too modestly. When it comes to the way you talk, it suggests you to not talk vulgarly or rudely yet not too academically when the circumstances don't call for it.

Now, a big modern-day challenge is how to integrate all six activities into the life of the average person in the 21st century. It seems to me that the most effective solution is to include those activities in the school program while also explaining their importance and their long-term benefits in our lives. A state of mind can be achieved in a personal way, but it can also be taught. So, it all starts at school, but it certainly doesn't end there.

Talking about the six necessary activities must take place elsewhere as well. And I believe it makes much sense to propose medical and healthcare centers. Doctors and medical practitioners should talk to all their patients about the six necessities, in addition to any prescribed medication or therapy. I said "all" patients, because it does apply to all patients, whether they have an infection-related issue or suffer from cancer or just frequent headaches or have harmless spots on their skin. This equally applies to a plethora of specialties, such as psychologists, life coaches, and dieticians.

You Want Information? Well, We Got Plenty! (Strike #1)

Furthermore, I want to stay on something truly remarkable for a moment. And that would be the tons, the scads, the overabundance of medical information that we managed to save from our ancestors. It is unbelievable how many understandable and accessible to the average person books we have from the past. Can you imagine the amount of information that we would have today if there had been no conflagrations nor pillages? But don't let me digress. I will focus on the positive side like I always try to do and recognize that it is part of our human nature to wish to leave something behind, to promote the science or sport or profession we love the most, to help others like us, and more generally, to make a change in any way we can; usually, a positive one.

Or Do You Want Similarities? Well, We Got Plenty Too! (Strike #2)

Aside from the knowledge abundance, studying writings of the medical field from the days of yore, one finds out pretty early in their research that — unexpectedly, perhaps — there are many similarities with the things we believe and practice to this day. From craniotomies to cauterization, it is pretty striking to find out how many common practices there are between ancient and modern medicine. Another very illustrating example is acupuncture. Nowadays, acupuncture has turned into a worldwide trend, with many TV shows and documentary series dedicating one of their episodes to it, yet it was developed in China approximately 4,000 years ago.

Prosthetics is another ancient idea. Today, replacing one's lost limbs with an artificial one is a no-brainer and a respectable number of athletes with artificial parts is admired around the world. In 2016, there were 4,342 athletes who took part in the fifteenth Summer Paralympic Games. Yet, the earliest prosthetic was discovered in Ancient Egypt, on a female mummy. Of course, in antiquity, the prosthetics were not functional; they were only used on people's dead bodies for esthetic purposes. That tells me that the necessary technological equipment wasn't there, but the conceptual idea was. And that's the most important thing. **Materialization is wonderful, but the idea is the only seed that can lead to it.** So, in brief, prosthetics is originally one of Ancient Egypt's brainchildren. We will meet them again later, by the way.

"WELLNESS": A NEW WORD FOR ANCIENT IDEAS

Before we move on, I would like to stay on the 'similarities' topic for a bit and mention tracheotomies, Caesarian sections (aka C-sections) – C-section is actually one of the oldest surgical operations – and, obviously, the broad use of herbs with medicinal properties. In antiquity, they were only used in the purest and most natural way, while presently, they are used either in a natural form or combined with something chemical. In the latter case, the herb constitutes the base of the final product. Finally, something that first appeared in antiquity is the Hippocratic Oath, the globally and wholly recognized oath for all medical professions.

And there are many other similarities between ancient and modern medical practice – make no mistake about that. As one would expect, a common ground between the two is the use of insect- or animal-derived products with medicinal properties. As one would also expect, the difference is that back then they were used in their pure form, whereas now we make use of fully-developed pharmaceutical products based on these natural elements. Those include ox bile, milk, honey, and cod liver oil, among others. In the past, they also used ants as a diuretic and to supply people suffering from anemia with blood. Today, we use ants' formic acid as a diuretic too. We also use lard, lanolin (wool fat of sheep), and beeswax as bases for various ointments, as our ancestors did. Another practice that has remained is taking a cold bath in case you have pyrexia, especially if your fever doesn't seem to drop. We still make use of Theophrastus' description concerning the extraction of tar from pine trees. Tar was then used on wound healing; now, it is still used on wound healing, but only for our tetrapod friends. Opium's special qualities were first observed and described by Hippocrates and Dioscorides and later on by Galen. Turpentine was and is used for coughs and lung complaints. Finally, splints, bandages, and even plaster cast are ancient inventions and not modern ones.

As for the differences between ancient and modern medicine, I think one of the major ones is the approach of the patient. More specifically, the turn taken nowadays is a more patient-centered approach called Functional Medicine. Functional Medicine addresses the patient as a whole (holistic approach) and not just an isolated set of symptoms. It engages both the patient and the practitioner in a therapeutic partnership. The latter listens to the histories of the former and observes the patient's interactions among genetic, environmental, and lifestyle factors that can influence long-term health and complex, chronic diseases. In our time and age, we fully acknowledge the role of psychology in any health situation and, by empowering patients to take an active role in their own health, Functional Medicine does just that.

Plenty of Forgotten Wisdom, As Well! (Strike #3)

Generally speaking, in the modern world, we have almost forgotten the health benefits of many superfoods known since antiquity. However, this tends to be turned around, as more and more studies remind us of the old days' simple life benefits, as more and more people feel unhappy in modern cities, as more and more patients grow desperate. Can anyone deny, though, that convenient foods, such as frozen pizzas and cheese doodles, have replaced healthy foods of the past, like many herbs, spices, and even homegrown vegetables? Sorry to break it to you, but **for every superfood that becomes a remnant of the past, we will pay the price with our health** — make no mistake about that.

Since humans began cooking over fire, bone broths from chicken, beef, fish or turkey meat were predominant in the traditional diet of not just the cultures that we are going to study here, but of every culture. And now this super superfood is sadly forgotten. We only think of it as the base for, say, soups, and that is all. Well, let's start with how to make bone broth, because the cooking method is what will lead us to its benefits. First, you roast the bones in the oven for several hours and then you boil the bones on the stove top for at least a day. Pretty simple, right? It might sound time-consuming, but think about it. It is time-consuming for your oven and not for you, really. So, it is that long cooking process breaking down the bones that releases key nutrients and unlocks many of the beneficial compounds inside the bones. But what is even more important is that this process makes them more digestible for us and allows easier assimilation of said key nutrients.

"WELLNESS": A NEW WORD FOR ANCIENT IDEAS

More precisely, they have protein-rich collagen that boosts skin strength, glucosamine which helps bone joints, chondroitin sulfate that helps rebuild cartilage, hyaluronic acid which is good for skin texture – us women know it well, – amino acids which are muscle boosters, and key minerals that can offer disease protection. Some of these benefits, we cannot get them from almost any other food. Add to that the benefits that we can get from the spices used in traditional recipes to cook it and you can see that bone broth is a really precious food that we should consider adding back into our diet even after all those centuries.

Turmeric, which we will meet again later, is one of those spices you should use when having bone broth and strengthen the health of your *entire* body. Ayurvedic herbalists, whom we will meet again as well, looked to turmeric for its health benefits. Its secret lies inside it and it is one of its compounds, called curcumin. The powerful antioxidant that is curcumin can help neutralize free radicals, alleviate joint discomfort, skin issues, and immune system challenges. Its antioxidant power can also prevent oxidation of LDL cholesterol molecules and some think that could explain why India, where turmeric is consumed on a daily basis, has some of the lowest rates of health challenges – especially heart disease – facing most of the Western world.

Later on in the book, we will see that each studied country had certain beliefs and superstitions of religious nature concerning diseases and sickness. Those national ideologies and superstitions are going to be presented individually as each country had its very own belief system. What I want to draw your attention on right now is that despite all those stumbling blocks that medicine faced, such as the impact of magical beliefs, religions, the presence of demons and other evil spirits, it still managed to be developed to an admirable degree and provide us with so much medical knowledge as if one of us had traveled in the past with a time machine and threatened them to prepare and write down all the basics of modern-day medicine and then some. Yes, their contribution is *that* important, and world-changing, and I will repeat what I said in the prologue: that I am deeply grateful to live in this time of constantly new marvelous discoveries.

FIRST PART OF THE JOURNEY: THE ASIAN TOUR

The first continent we are going to visit will be the largest one, that is Asia. And we are going to stay there for a while because we have three stops to make: China, India, and Iran. Again, I have preferred the alphabetical order, since I do not want to comment on their importance by listing them in order of evolution and progress; well, at least not yet. I will probably leave that for the last chapter of my study where the various conclusions will be taking over.

It is true that even today many people quickly associate traditional Chinese herbal remedies and acupuncture with Eastern alternative medicine and nothing more. Especially in the West, Chinese medicine is seen as the ur-alternative to the dominating industrialized medicine. For some, it is just a little more worthwhile than charlatanism, attributing its successes to the placebo effect and the odd folk remedy. But this is not the case; they are just largely unfamiliar with other medical practices established across the Asian continent. Traditional Chinese Medicine (aka TCM) is the best-known Asian medical practice around the world and is closely associated with the ideas of wellness and wellbeing, which are the ultimate goals. The Indian and Iranian contributions are exceptionally significant as well, but overall the contribution in the progress of the medical science within the Asian continent does not end there.

Not wishing to be not even a little unfair to anyone, I would like to use my "Asian" introduction for briefly mentioning another four civilizations that are truly worthy of a medicophile's attention. Firstly,

"WELLNESS": A NEW WORD FOR ANCIENT IDEAS

there is Bhutan and its gSo-ba Rig-Pa (that is, the science of healing). The basic principle in Bhutanese medicine is to balance the three principal energies of the body. The medical practitioner employs the ancient tools of pulse diagnosis and urine analysis to find the root causes of their patient's disease. The treatment is carried out through all the usual suspects, that is diet changes, lifestyle adjustments, and herbal medicines grown naturally in Bhutan and the Himalayas. For those of you who may not know, Bhutan is a sovereign state located in the Eastern Himalayas in South Asia. It borders two of our journey's stops: China to the north and India to the south, east and west. Therefore, it is easy to understand why all three countries had a noteworthy medical contribution; as for many other things in life, communication is the key in this case too. I should also mention that Bhutanese medicine is primarily based upon the Buddhist principles and the close relationship between mind and body.

Secondly, there is Vietnam and its notable medical progress. The distinguish feature of Traditional Vietnamese Medicine (TVM) is its emphasis on nourishing the blood and vital energy, rather than concentrating on specific symptoms, as happens in other civilizations' medicine. For TVM, the key to good health is building up the blood (e.g. after loss) and energy in the human body. The main treatments employed by TVM are acupuncture, moxibustion, and herbal medicine. The first two will be explicitly analyzed later. Moxibustion is not as popular as acupuncture, but even if you think you are familiar with the latter, there are definitely certain characteristics that are wrongly perceived by the majority. The pillar of the TVM theories is based on the observed effects of the body's qi (energy). Qi can be inherited from the parents or extracted from our food. Once again, all you need to know about qi is included later on in this study. Another TVM cornerstone is the blood and the "fuel" gathered and stored by our body. It is true that TVM evolved together with TCM and the development of the two is so intertwined that they have many identical parts.

Thirdly, there is Japan and its developed herbal medicine, which has a long history of clinical application. It is called Kampo and it consists of precisely measured herbs for the treatment of illnesses. A distinguished feature of Kampo is that it does not use products made from rare or even endangered plant or animal species, so it is followed by no protest whatsoever about such malpractices. Another one is that it is based on a popularly accepted theory: that diseases arise due to a disharmony in the flow of the aforementioned qi. In the second place, it is based on the skillful use of well-known formulas, valued for their impact and effectiveness not only on clearly described but (almost) equally on vaguely described conditions. Concerning prevention, Kampo suggests its patients to follow natural principles in order to maintain their good health.

And fourthly, there is Korea and its traditional medicine, which will be referred to as TKM. Originating centuries ago, TKM is an ancient practice of healing that does not just cure locally an illness or ailment, but deals with the whole body; it is a form of medicine that treats holistically. It certainly has several overlaps with the medicine of other countries, such as China, India, and Japan, the most evident (and popular as well) being acupuncture. TKM is based on the Eastern philosophy. The human body is viewed as a miniature version of the universe. The principles, treatment methods and medication for the physiology and pathology of the body are explained by the Yin-Yang and the Five Elements theories. TKM does not attempt to learn about the body by dissection, experimentation or analysis, but instead observes natural bodily functions as they appear in order to diagnose an illness or ailment. It also never limits the cause of even the most minor ailment to a local one, but examines the entire body to find the reason for the condition. By correcting the bodily imbalance rather than performing surgery or other invasive procedure, it adopts a natural-cure approach. In other words, TKM does not just treat the side effects created by the illness, but seeks to discover its cause, which is then either eliminated or improved. As such, it is virtually impossible to summarize the principles and philosophy of TKM in a single word or sentence or to really have a logical understanding of it.

The many negations used in the previous paragraph were not accidental. I talked about the differences between the philosophy and approach of medical issues of each country or civilization and the challenges that they create. So, those negations were used to demonstrate exactly that. And they were used at the very end of — as I like to call it — my Asian introduction to make sure that they stick with the reader right from the beginning of the analysis of the five wisely chosen traditional medicines.

BALANCE: THE ONE TO OPEN OUR EYES IS CHINA!

▌ The History of Traditional Chinese Medicine

As expected, China's history of medicine is a long one. Chinese medicine had an early start. It is an ancient medical system based on the Daoist view of a universe where everything is interrelated. The Traditional Chinese Medicine (which will only be referred to as TCM from now on, to save precious time and space) offers a unique and truly astonishing method of understanding the structure of our internal organs and our body's physiological processes. It has been developed by the Chinese medical practitioners through thousands of years of observation and practice. It is a natural, holistic medicinal system, still practiced throughout the world today. And this is exactly what fascinates me more than anything; that an ancient practice is still used by millions of people all over the world, even after the development of modern scientific and technological medicine.

So, having passed the test of modern medicine, it is safe to say that TCM truly has withstood that coveted test of time. The documented history of TCM dates back more than 4,000 years to the times of *Shennong* (Yan Emperor), while mature TCM theory was established during the Song dynasty (960-1279 AD). TCM theory is based on a holistic, interconnected view of the world. As we will see, the patient is considered as a system in which the normal balance of Yin-Yang has been disrupted; thus, the disease is that Yin-Yang imbalance. However, I would like to point out that in the People's Republic of China, the term

"WELLNESS": A NEW WORD FOR ANCIENT IDEAS

"TCM" is one that was given in the late 1970s to the healthcare ideas and practices generated between 1950 and 1975. So, apart from numerous influences, the term TCM has nothing to do with medicines and therapies within the ancient Chinese medical system.

Dr. Paul Unschuld has spoken repeatedly and explicitly of the matter and he has established a distinction between TCM and CTM (that is, Chinese traditional medicine). This way, he gets to mean the same thing as the Chinese people with the term TCM and he proposes the use of the term CTM to refer to the entire body of knowledge accumulated in the millennia before the advent of the 20th century. Now, much as I would like to set the record straight like I always try to do, the acronym TCM (following the word order Traditional Chinese Medicine) is way too established on a global scale for me to overturn.

At the beginnings of the Bronze Age, China had its first proper civilization during the Shang Dynasty (1600-1046 BC). Writing was already developed and they adored a deity called Shangdi (or simply Di), who lived in heaven along with all dead ancestors. The worship of their ancestors was and still is very important in China. At the time, it was believed that illness resulted from upsetting an ancestor and consequently being cursed by them. Therefore, since an evil demon had entered the patient's body, curing them involved bringing peace back to the upset ancestor through the appropriate ritual or asking for the ancestor's help to expel the evil demon. This was part of the Ancient Chinese Shamanistic medicine.

Shamans were mediators who talked to the ancestors, who in turn talked to Shangdi. They asked questions by writing them on "oracle bones." These were usually scapula bones or tortoise shells, which they heated afterwards and their cracks were "divined," that is, read by a shaman in order to get an answer. To discover ancient history, we rely on archeological finds and writings. Bronze was a very expensive material and, so, what was written in this era was the possessions of the rich (ritual bronzes and shells). As a consequence, we cannot know the (probably very interesting) remedies and medicines that the simple folk used, since they were neither wealthy nor educated. In some regions of the East, such as Vietnam and Tibet, shamanistic medicine survived almost intact.

Then came the Zhou Dynasty (1046-249 BC), certainly a high point in the history of Chinese civilization. However, during the Spring and Autumn Period (770-476) of the Eastern Zhou Period (770-221), centralized power control declined, the local aristocracy started to fight among themselves, and social order degenerated into the Warring States Period (476-221), a time of great instability. However, it was those unstable times that produced great thinkers, such as Confucius who was born in 551 BC. Different philosophies dating back into antiquity were studied for possible solutions to problems of the present. This was the era of the "Hundred Schools of Thought" and thankfully, much was recorded during that time.

The major medical body of work was the Huangdi Neijing (*The Yellow Emperor's Inner Classic of Medicine*, sometimes incorrectly translated as "The Yellow Emperor's Classic of Internal Medicine"). It was drawn up during the Hundred Schools period (3rd century BC) incorporating most of the earlier discovered knowledge. This body of work is the earliest one describing in depth the practice and theoretical underpinnings of what clearly is acupuncture in the modern sense, that is, the manipulation of qi or vapors flowing in vessels or conduits by means of needling. You can liken it to a sort of encyclopedia.

It is a compilation of much earlier – Huangdi is said to have lived in the 3rd millennium BC – material, enriched with added commentaries; besides, the Chinese are notorious for their love for commentary writing. Concerning the content of the book, I myself would also like to add a comment of mine; I find it noteworthy that surgery is only mentioned as a last medical resort, like in the case of tumor removing.

The thing is that there is no historical reference to a text by this name until the late first century BC, and that book may or may not have been a version of one of the surviving texts. Interestingly, the information presented in the Huangdi Neijing is not necessarily even Chinese in origin. You see, Huangdi's minister Qi Bo (or Qi Po) is an enigmatic figure. Some sources present him as a mythological Chinese doctor who was enlightened with the knowledge of TCM by an ethereal being from the heavens. However, most scholars believe that Qi Bo existed. The German academic Dr. Paul U. Unschuld, who is the West's leading authority on ancient Chinese healing practices, has a particular view on the subject. Unschuld has spent decades of his life studying and translating with scrupulousness Chinese and ancient Chinese medical texts. He has also collected 1,100 antique manuscripts that could give clues to how medicine was practiced at China's grass-roots level. In his spare time, Dr. Unschuld has led German government delegations to China, and has written books on how medicine helps to explain China's rise to global prominence. Based on the fact that Qi Bo has no background in Chinese history or mythology, coupled with the phonetic resemblances of the two names (the Han-period pronunciation of Qi Bo's name was *G'ieg Pak*), Unschuld was led to believe that Qi Bo might actually have been Hippocrates of Cos. He suggests that the name Qi Bo may be a Chinese approximation of Hippocrates. The ideogram Qi means "mountain path" and the ideogram Po means "white man", so Qi and Po together means "The white man who came from the mountain path". This probably refers to somebody from the West, as China only has mountains in the west. The German academic has also found a few more lexical comparisons between Ancient Greek and Chinese for the words for thirst (*dipsa*, in Greek – xiao ke, in Chinese), phthisis (fei xiao), and cholera (huo luan). It is likely that in China, just as on the Indian subcontinent, transregional flows of knowledge, technology, and people played a significant role.

Moving on, the Han Dynasty (206 BC-220 AD) is considered a golden age in Chinese history. During the Han years, there were many medical discoveries. This was the time when people thought of illnesses as an imbalance between the yin and the yang, an imbalance that destroys the body's wellness and the soul's wellbeing. This was the time when many different curing techniques, such as acupuncture and moxibustion, were put into extended practice. And, finally, this was the time when the Chinese made a crucial discovery about the human body. They found out that when you listen to an individual's heartbeat or feeling their pulse, you can tell whether they are healthy or not. An analysis of terms, like the yin and yang theory, acupuncture, and moxibustion is certainly called for. However, not wanting to stop the historical flow here in the beginning, we will discuss them later on.

Following the Han Dynasty, the next great age in China concerning the progress of medicine was the Tang Dynasty (618-907 AD) preceded by the worth-mentioning Sui Dynasty (581-618 AD). The first Tang emperor was the founder of the first medical school in China, established in 629 AD. In 657, another Tang emperor (Gaozong) commissioned the literary project of publishing an official *materia medica* featuring an official classification of all the medicines used in pharmacology. More than 800 medicinal substances are mentioned, taken from various metals, minerals, stones, plants, herbs, animals, vegetables, fruits, and cereal crops. During that era, it was firstly identified in writing that patients with diabetes had an excess of sugar in their urine and it was recognized that they should avoid consuming alcohol and foods with starch.

The Golden Chamber of Chang Chung-Ching

Regarded as one of the great physicians of the Han dynasty, the most glorious period in Chinese medical history, Chang Chung-Ching (Zhang Zhongjing) wrote the 'Treatise on Febrile and Other Diseases (*Shang Han Za Bing Lun*). This treatise had a profound influence on Chinese medicine and is considered an important medical classic. It included over one hundred effective herbal formulas, many of them still in use today, and other formulas, such as the gynecological remedy Tang-kuei and Peony formula (called Danggui Shaoyao San) which is today applied to disorders during pregnancy, post-partum weakness, infertility, and prevention of miscarriage. His work called 'Synopsis of Prescriptions of the Golden Chamber' (Jinkui Yaolue Fanglun) is of comparable importance and also still in print. The entirety of his writings has been the subject of much study, numerous commentaries, and improved editions. Chang Chung-Ching paid close attention to the physical signs, symptoms, kind and course of a disease and he stood for the dignity and responsibility of the medical profession. All that led to him being called the Hippocrates of China.

"WELLNESS": A NEW WORD FOR ANCIENT IDEAS

The Prolific Sun Simiao

Sun Simiao was a renowned TCM doctor of the Sui and Tang dynasties. He practiced preserving health through qigong. Sun was the author of the earliest Chinese encyclopedia of clinical practice and was titled as China's King of Medicine for his significant contributions to Chinese medicine and painstaking care to his patients. Equally, he was worshipped as the Medicine Buddha, a deity invoked during healing practices. He recorded his experience with herb formulas and his knowledge of medicine in his famous 30-volume work called "Prescriptions for Emergencies Worth a Thousand Gold" and printed in 652 AD. This body of work presented life-saving remedies, hence the title showing the great value. It covers a broad range of categories--from basic medical theories to different clinical subjects, and from theories and methodologies to prescription formulas and drugs. It also covers materials from the classics in one segment, while another category includes the empirical formulas and prescriptions that were circulated among the populace. This book included the strong points of different schools and is suitable for people from different educational backgrounds. It was a treatise on medical practice that reviewed the work since the Han Dynasty, beginning with the concepts of the *Neijing*. In it, he included treatises on acupuncture, moxibustion, massage, diet, and exercises. He emphasized the importance of gathering herbs at the right time and he insisted that herbs must be fresh and come from the genuine source. It is only logical that it remains popular and plays a guiding role even to this day.

Sun Simiao's second book, printed in 682 AD, was a supplement to his first one. Its content was based on thirty years of subsequent experience with special attention given to folk remedies. This work of 30 volumes also serves as a *Materia Medica* with 800 medicinal materials, providing details about the collection and preparation of 200 of them. He presented some new herbs, especially ones from foreign countries, notably from India, the source of the Buddhist tradition that he pursued. Two volumes were devoted to study of the formulas and treatment strategies of the Shanghan Lun (circa 220 AD).

In addition, the supplement presented about 2,000 more formulas, though these have not been studied and retained by future generations to the extent of the formulas from the first book. The second book also included considerable references to mystical and magical practices, such as exorcisms. He mentioned 32 drugs that were said to be effective against demons, and he carefully described the thirteen acupuncture points, that were known as the demon-releasing points. The last two volumes included talismans, amulets, and incantations. Both of Sun's books are still reprinted today, compiled as one under the title Qianjin Fang.

Sun Simiao authored over 80 books in his lifetime; books that passed onto future generations and made him the larger than life person that he was. But what interests us more in the context of this study is his vast contribution to medicine and his outstanding medical ethics. He expressed his belief that medicine is an art of kindness, which really is a very moving thing to say. In his book *Sincerity and Devotion of Great Doctors*, he wrote that doctors must be concentrated, calm, free of desires and pursuits, and treat their patients indiscriminately. He clearly had a noble character as a doctor. Sun adopted a holistic approach to treating illnesses. He believed that by skillful nursing and recuperating successfully, one could be free of illnesses. Sun Simiao valued preserving health and actively practiced it. Because he was good at the art of cultivating health, he lived to over 100 and still enjoyed good vision and hearing when he was old.

He combined ideas on the preservation of health from Confucianism and Taoism, as well as from ancient India, with those of TCM. He proposed many practical and effective ways to cultivate good health, which, even now, guide people's daily lives. Sun was also the first to invent a urethral catheter. According to historical records, one of his patients could not pass urine. Seeing that the patient was in extreme pain, Sun thought he should use some kind of tube into his urethra and make the urine flow out naturally, since it was too late to treat that patient with medicines. The "tube" he used to give it a try was a green onion stem, which is very thin, long, and soft. Having chosen a suitable green onion stem, he charred it gently, cut the sharp end off, and then carefully inserted it into the patient's urethra. He then blew into the tube once. As expected, the urine flew out of the tube. The patient's bloated abdomen gradually became smaller, and his illness was also cured.

His first book gave special attention to the treatment of women and children, with the first three volumes devoted to women's disorders, including pregnancy and post-partum disorders, and the next two about diseases of infants and breast-feeding. The famous Song Dynasty specialists in gynecology, obstetrics, and pediatrics, who influenced all subsequent work on these scientific subjects, relied upon Sun's work as their basis.

By cultivating morality and the body with virtue and by having both virtue and talent, Sun Simiao became a great figure whom common people and medical professionals for several generations have highly respected. He is considered the first to have presented issues related to ethics of medical treatment, depicting the characteristics of a great physician and cautioning other physicians about developing behavior that was inappropriate to their serious and respectable profession.

Sun Simiao is probably best known for his intense interest in the identification and preparation of herbs and his definitive work with formulation principles. His formulas, either the purgative or the chill- or wind-dispelling or even the cough-relieving ones present a particular interest due to the variety of their ingredients. Indicatively, his Croton and Hematite Formula consisted of croton, hematite, apricot seed, and kaolin, and was used to alleviate constipation, to purge fluids, and to lower rising qi. His Tang-kuei Combination Formula consisted of tang-kuei, cinnamon, zanthoxylum, dry ginger, licorice, pinellia, magnolia bark, ginseng, astragalus, and peony; it was used for cold spleen or stomach with pain in the chest and abdomen. His aforementioned special attention to the treatment of women and children led to a number of pregnancy and post-partum formulas, such as the *Zhuli Tang* Formula, made with bamboo sap, siler, scute, ophiopogon, and hoelen, that was used to treat irritability and restlessness during pregnancy.

TCM was carefully designed to promote and help maintain health through proper diet and physical exercise. Any ailment, illness or disease is treated with either acupuncture, herbs, or qi gong – all of which will be properly analyzed; don't you worry — or a combination of those. As I said, Chinese medicine practitioners diagnose and treat all types of sickness, with TCM being an undeniably valid and effective form of medicine. At the root of TCM, we find the belief that the individual, which is the microcosm, is viewed as an integral part of the forces of nature, which is the macrocosm. It is based on a set of interventions designed to restore the absolute balance in each individual. Carefully observing the nature, Daoist sages were able to perceive patterns that are common to both the external environment and the internal "climate" of the human body. These cumulative observations of sages all over China has led to the birth of that intricately intricate system of diagnosis and healing with the acronym TCM.

Daoism: Yet Another Influential Factor on Medicine

Of course, traditional systems of medicine also exist in other South and East Asian countries, such as Japan and Korea. As expected once again, these systems have been influenced by TCM and have many elements in common, but each system has certainly developed its own distinctive features. Now, back to TCM, which has its roots in the ancient philosophy of Daoism and dates back more than 2,500 years. It originated in the region of Eastern Asia which today includes China, Tibet, Vietnam, Korea, and Japan. Contrary to what many people might think, Daoism is not a religion. Nor is it a medical sector. It is a philosophy (based on the concept of Dao) that had a strong influence on medicine. Your next two questions will probably be "which is the concept of Dao?" and "which is Daoism's influence on medicine?". I will answer them implicitly, that is briefly but sufficiently as always, and then we will get back to the complex TCM system again. You probably noticed that I use a D where most people would use a T in terms, such as Dao, Daoism, Daoist et cetera. Well, when I write something — whether it is an essay, a study, or whatever else, — apart from giving poignantly my point of view, I also want to set the record straight when I see that it is needed. And in this case, I felt that need. The spelling difference is a translation from Chinese to English issue. For a period of time, the

"WELLNESS": A NEW WORD FOR ANCIENT IDEAS

West translated the Chinese D as T. More recently, though, this switched back to D. In conclusion, using a Delightful D is more au-courant and sophisticated than using a Tired-old T, and, being the nonconformist that I am, that is exactly what I am going to do.

So, Dao (or, somewhat erroneously, Tao) means "the way" and is the mother of all the phenomena that we know. Before Dao, there was chaos; and Dao was then manifested as the universe, something unimaginable, unknown and unknowable. It is the eternal primeval law of nature and is expressed through the duality of the Yin and the Yang, which we will study later on. All in all, you can say that Dao is something comparable to today's "big bang" theory. I know you were thinking it! So, one objective of TCM is to keep yin and yang, these mutually dependent and polar opposites at the same time, in harmonious balance within a person. In addition to yin and yang, Daoist teachers believed that the Dao also produced a third force, a primordial energy or qi (sometimes spelled as chi or ki in English, as well). The interplay between yin, yang, and qi gave rise to the Five Elements, that is, water, metal, earth, wood, and fire. These entities are all reflected somehow in the structure and functioning of the human body.

Its influence on medicine has to do with the way people conduct themselves throughout the different seasons of a year. The idea of humans being part of nature and needing to remain in harmony with it was fundamental ("As above, so below"). In particular, in the wintertime, one should go to bed early and get up late, without wasting too much energy, because winter (time of strong Yin) is the time of conservation and storage, while in the summertime, one should rise early and go to bed late, because summer (time of strong Yang) is the time to be outdoors and it is when people naturally have more energy to expend. This way, not only the weather changes but equally people's behavior come full circle within a year.

Treatment Methods

The treatment methods that are included under the general heading of TCM are numerous, such as acupuncture, moxibustion, therapeutic exercise, massage, various herbal remedies, dietary regulation, and other therapeutic practices. These forms of treatments are largely based upon beliefs way different from the disease concept favored by Western medicine practices. So, what is referred to as disease or sickness or illness in the West, is considered to be a matter of disharmony or imbalance in TCM. One thing that makes TCM so complex is the fact that it encompasses the dogmas of many philosophies. It is heavily rooted in traditional Eastern philosophies; plural. There was no one single philosophy and did not originate in only one era of Chinese history, obviously. TCM is based on an intricate philosophy that was built on, added to, and modified throughout the centuries. This is very typical of the Chinese, who are a very pragmatic people, among other characteristics. They have no problem accepting a wide variety of philosophies into their culture and not seeing any conflict between them. More precisely, the philosophy behind Chinese medicine is a melding of tenets from Buddhism, Confucianism and Daoism, aka The Three Teachings, which coexisted harmoniously in China.

As a result of this blend, many schools of thought were formed among TCM practitioners, though naturally its basis is common and it is formed by the following five Daoist axioms:

1. There are natural laws that govern the entire universe, including human beings.
2. The natural order of the universe is innately harmonious and well-organized. When people live according to the laws of the universe, they live in harmony with that universe and the natural environment.
3. The universe is dynamic, with change being its only constant element. Stagnation is in opposition to the law of the universe and causes (what Western medicine calls) illness.
4. All living things are interconnected and interdependent.
5. Humans are intimately connected to and affected by all facets of their environment.

The Humble Confucius

Confucius was born at the end of the Eastern Zhou period (and at the beginning of the Warring States period). We have learned about him from the Analects, a collection of sayings and ideas attributed to him and his contemporaries, written by his disciples. Confucius wanted to be a monarch's advisor. He traveled around in search of a monarch that would give him the credit he was looking for, but no one wanted his ideas; he was too moral. All the monarchic leaders preferred pragmatic techniques to use and win wars. So, he became a teacher in the end. His ideas were taken seriously two whole centuries after his death! He talked about humbleness, modesty, humility, honor, respect, gentlemanlike behavior, and moderation. The Confucian idea of moderation is apparent in the Neijing in several passages. He stressed that health can be maintained if people's lifestyle is characterized by moderation and not excessiveness. Seeing that he lived during a warful period, he was occupied with the dealing of soldiers, as well. He accentuated that a wise person would not treat those who have already fallen sick, but rather those who are not yet sick. So, he introduced indirectly the idea of medical prevention in his own way.

The Five Elements Theory

Ancient Greek medical practitioners learned about the structures of the human body from dissection. By contrast, traditional Chinese physicians built up an understanding of the location and functions of the major human organs over centuries of observation, because they believed that cutting open a body insulted the individual's ancestors. Therefore, we can see crystal clear the influence of religion on medicine and medical practice. Then, Chinese physicians correlated the organs with their principles of yin, yang, qi, and the Five Elements. Thus, wood is related to the liver (yin) and the gall bladder (yang); fire is associated with the heart (yin) and the small intestine (yang); earth is related to the spleen (yin) and the stomach (yang); metal to the lungs (yin) and the large intestine (yang); and, finally, water to the kidneys (yin) and the bladder (yang). Moreover, the Chinese believed that the body contains Five Essential Substances, which include blood, spirit, vital essence (a principle of growth and development produced by the body from the combination of qi and blood); fluids (all body fluids other than blood, such as saliva, spinal fluid, sweat, etc.); and qi.

Another element that is unique to TCM is the **meridian system.** Chinese medical practitioners considered the body to be a network of multiple energy pathways called meridians. The meridians link and balance the various human organs. They have the following four functions: to connect the internal organs with the exterior of the body and, by extension, connect the person to the environment and the universe; to harmonize the yin and yang principles within the body's organs and the Five Substances; to distribute qi within the body; and to protect the body against external imbalances related to weather (wind, summer heat, dampness, dryness, cold, and fire).

The earliest known Chinese medical text is "The Recipes for Fifty-Two Ailments" and it was written about 186 BC. These "recipes" suggest chanting spells, various herbal medicines, lancing (that is, cutting the skin open), and cauterization (that is, controlled burning of the flesh) as cures for situations like warts, snake bites, and possession by demons (that is, what we would call "mental illness" today). By the time of the Han Dynasty, about 100 BC, China had already become a major center of medical research, which also meant that some of the world's best physicians worked there. Which, in turn, resulted in the writing of a historic book about medicine, called "Neijing." In this book, you could find organized and explained all the treatments of those physicians.

According to the Neijing, earlier ideas about demons making you sick were wrong, while the imbalance between the yin and the yang was given as the explanation of illnesses. Indicatively, lifestyle choices, such as bad-quality diet, lack of exercise, too much stress, and other environmental factors, can knock somebody out of balance and block their qi, their life force, something like Herophilos's idea of *pneuma* (spirit). Like Herophilos did in Egypt — the fourth stop in our journey — 300 years earlier, at least one Han Dynasty physician dissected a dead person, about 23 AD, in order to discover a little bit more about the human body. Another Han Dynasty physician, named Huo Tuo, apparently combined wine and hashish to use as an anesthetic for surgery. Regrettably, the medical books that Huo Tuo wrote have all been lost. It is possible that he got medical information from Buddhist missionaries from India – the second stop in our journey. Chinese physicians were also influenced by Greek ideas, such as the four humors theory, travelling along the Silk Road. I think it is quite evident how much interconnected our five stops are; besides, four of them were mentioned in this very paragraph.

It is fascinating that many similar traditional practices and ideas were believed around Eurasia at about the same time. For example, Wu Xing aka the Five Elements aka the Five Phases is a traditional concept noticeably similar to the Greek scientific ideas of the Five Elements – earth, water, air, fire, and ether – that date from before Socrates and remain widely believed by Europeans until modern times. This concept is also similar to the ancient Indian and Buddhist ideas of the Four Elements – the same ones, minus ether.

It is true that Chinese physicians figured out many ways to treat sick people. They used many medicines made of different herbs and tree barks. Though some of them were just guesses, other medicines worked fairly well. By the 300s AD, Ge Hong was the first medical practitioner in the world to write a good medicine for malaria. Physicians in China also learned from Indian physicians about the practice of inoculation against smallpox, and by the 1500s AD, under the Ming Dynasty, Chinese physicians were inoculating many people to prevent smallpox from spreading.

Our Beloved Acupuncture

Let's now study the different TCM treatment forms. I am going to begin with acupuncture, which is probably the most familiar one worldwide. We already know that it is often used for pain relief, however, in traditional Chinese practice, it certainly has wider applications. It is closely connected to the body's overall wellness and eudemonia and it's based upon a notion that views the meridians as conduits or pathways for the qi, that is, the energy of life. According to this notion, disease is attributed to an obstruction of the meridians. Acupuncture is then used to treat any affliction of our internal organs as well as muscular and skin issues. It involves the practice of inserting fine needles, usually no thicker than a human hair, into the skin.

The insertion of needles at specific points along the meridians is believed to unblock the qi. More than 800 acupuncture points have been identified, but only about fifty are commonly used. Chinese medicine theory holds that there are meridians or channels in our body, through which energy flows. These channels serve as connections between the Zang Fu organs and all the other structures of the body, so the free flow of energy through them helps maintain health. All acupuncture points have local effects and are useful for treating pain or dysfunction in a given area. Some acupuncture points, however, have general effects on the body as a whole.

For example, one of the most familiar acupuncture points is ST 36, which can be used either to tonify the qi or to break up blood stasis in the chest. The effects of acupuncture points depend not only on the function of the points, but also on the way they are needled and on the depth at which they are needled. There are, obviously, numerous needling techniques and variations and there is a recommended depth for needling, too. So, going back to the ST 36 point, if the point is needled at a moderate depth, then the needling technique is one of gentle qi tonification; if the point is needled more deeply and a strong sedating or dispersing technique is used, then the blood stasis in the chest can successfully be broken up. So, it is of utmost importance that an acupuncture practitioner has mastered not only the location of the points, but equally the knowledge of appropriate needling techniques and depths of insertion.

Since we are studying acupuncture at length, I would like to name a few more techniques that can be used to affect acupuncture points. No, needles are not the only way, as most of us thought. There is also the suction cup method; there are also massage techniques known as Tui Na that may be used; or a few drops of blood may be taken from said points. And there are also a few variations if we do use needles.

"WELLNESS": A NEW WORD FOR ANCIENT IDEAS

For example, electrical stimulation may be applied to the needle or a special herb called moxa may be burned on the needle over the point to heat it up. This variation is called moxibustion, it is pretty useful, and we will revisit it later on. The use of the aforementioned techniques depends on the symptoms of the patient and the overall pattern of disharmony of that individual.

There are studies upon studies on how and why acupuncture works; all of them inadequate and inconclusive. There is still no consensus on the mechanism behind it. However, the National Institutes of Health (NIH), in the USA, has reached to the "halfway" consensus that acupuncture is an effective treatment for several disorders and that further research is necessary. Well, judging by the ever-growing interest in Chinese medicine within the Western scientific community, I believe that future studies will be able to provide even more insight. Besides, there are already fourteen studies having shown that acupuncture and hypnosis are promising alternatives to smoking-cessation drugs for people who are trying to quit smoking. Apparently, acupuncture triggers the release of feel-good hormones that can help alleviate withdrawal symptoms, while hypnosis can induce an altered mental state allowing one to concentrate on breaking their bad habit.

Of course, ancient acupuncture is not an exclusive possession of the Chinese. The papyrus Ebers from 1550 BC is the most important of the Ancient Egyptian medical treaties. It refers to a book on the subject of vessels which could correspond to the twelve meridians of acupuncture. Equally, the Bantu (in South Africa) sometimes scratch parts of the patient's body to cure a disease. In the treatment of sciatica, the Bantu cauterize a part of the ear using a hot metal probe. This practice corresponds to the acupuncture method of Auricular or Ear acupuncture. Some Eskimos practice a simple type of acupuncture using sharp stones, just like in ancient Chinese acupuncture. In an isolated tribe in Brazil, people shoot tiny arrows with a blowpipe into specific parts of the body. All in all, the great contribution of the Chinese to the primitive, or largely local form of acupuncture practices mentioned above, is that they have developed a fairly complete systemic method.

In fact, archaeological excavations in sites all around China in the last century have brought to light a number of pointed stones which archaeologists have determined to be ancient acupuncturing needles. Those stones were used for various medical treatments, such as making skin incisions or stimulating specific points of the body. After the stones, they used slivers of animal bones and later on, needles made of bamboo. Another excavation at a site from the Shang period revealed a stone hook which was contained in a lacquer casket and used as a medical instrument in ancient Chinese acupuncture. But it is not only those needles and instruments that demonstrate acupuncture's special place in the heart of Ancient China. There was also a bronze statue at the size of a man created to show the acupuncture points on the human body. The famous acupuncturist Wang Wei-Yi, who created the Bronze Acupuncture Statue, also compiled a book called *Tongren Zhenjiu Shuxue Tujing* (Illustrated Canon of Acupuncture Points based upon the Bronze Figure). According to the book *Songshi* (History of the Song Dynasty), Emperor Renzong, who got sick in 1034, was successfully cured with the use of acupuncture. Obviously, this helped make acupuncture more popular, while medical practitioners actually began to become specialized in this method.

Catalogued and described in many textbooks, acupuncture is taught at universities and is reproducible under experimental conditions. The methods and practice of acupuncture have come a long way since its humble ancient beginnings, but the interest and desire to understand this ancient art remains as fresh as ever. Lastly, acupuncture is usually used as a treatment in combination with herbal remedies, so the latter will be the second TCM feature we are going to study.

Herbal Medicine

Chinese herbal remedies differ from Western herbalism in several respects. In Chinese practice, they are used according to each plant's effect on an individual's qi and the Five Elements. TCM uses many formulas to treat certain common imbalance patterns, formulas that can be modified to correspond to the needs of every person more accurately. Herbs are carefully selected, processed, and dried. They are given to a patient in a tea or pill, or in the form of pharmaceutical grade extracts. The latter is the growing choice for most patients and practitioners. A typical TCM herbal formula contains four classes of ingredients, arranged in a hierarchical order. There has to be a chief (the principal ingredient, chosen for the patient's specific illness), a deputy (to reinforce the chief's action or treat a coexisting condition), an assistant (to counteract side effects of the first two ingredients), and finally an envoy (to harmonize all the other ingredients and convey them to the parts of the body that they are to treat).

The basic principle of Chinese herbal medicine is the combination of individual herbs into formulas that will promote one's health. There are literally thousands of herbs used medicinally, though about 400 of them are commonly used. Common Chinese herbal medicines include astragalus root, reishi mushroom, goji berry, ginkgo biloba, ginseng, and others. After a practitioner uncovers the disharmony pattern underlying a complaint of the patient, an individualized herbal formula is constructed to correct this pattern. Sometimes, only a single herb is used; however, combinations of herbs into complex formulas are more commonly applied. Individualized herbal formulas are typically based on a classical formula for the pattern, but they may also be based on modern clinical trials. Individual herbs are then subtracted or added to the combination to fit the patient's needs as accurately as possible and to treat all symptoms. This flexibility allows for a more targeted treatment approach.

Formulas typically contain between five and fifteen herbs. The art of devising an herbal formula is complex and takes years to master. Centuries of tradition have categorized each herb in terms of its taste, temperature (whether it warms or cools the body), and the Meridians and Zang Fu organs it affects. Each herb also has contraindications and specific doses that must be taken into account. Finally, herbs interact with each other in various ways, some helping, and others antagonizing each other. Therefore, it is important that a practitioner prescribing herbs have a comprehensive understanding about all of this information and how it affects a particular pattern of disharmony.

Likewise, there can be interactions between Chinese herbs and conventional medication, so it is important that patients be monitored for side effects and followed to see whether the formula is effective. Depending on the condition, herbal formulas may be changed every 3 days to once a month. Besides being ingested in tablet or liquid form, specific herbal formulas may also be used as an external application, as an enema, or as a douche. Much like the choice of herbs and formula, the mode of application is dependent on the nature of the disorder and the most effective means of treatment. Nowadays, an herbalist oftentimes works closely with a physician to manage a patient's treatment, especially if the herbal therapy can or might interact with the patient's prescription medications.

The main thing I would like to point out with this study is how "contemporary" these analyzed "ancient" medical practices actually are, so I could not leave out a 2002 study in Texas which showed that a traditional Chinese anti-rheumatic herb extract helped patients with rheumatoid arthritis by improving symptoms, such as morning stiffness and tender, swollen joints. Its side effects (decreased appetite and nausea) were tolerable for those aided by the herb. Another scientific study of the same year showed that there are new benefits to applying soy proteins, an ancient Chinese practice, to the skin. A new form of soy proteins preparation showed benefits, among other things, in reducing age spots and ultraviolet ray damage, and smoothing and moisturizing the skin.

Have You Heard of Moxibustion?

Apart from being an intriguing-sounding word, moxibustion is an externally applied TCM treatment which consists of burning dried mugwort (aka moxa aka *Artemisia argyi*), a small and spongy herb, on particular points on the body to facilitate healing. Mugwort is compressed and rolled into cigar-shaped herbal sticks which are then lit and held over acupuncture points. Moxibustion is thought to send heat and nourishing qi into the body. So, it is really a form of heat therapy. It has a dual effect of fortification and purgation in TCM theories, which are based on the actions of the meridian system and the roles of moxa and fire. It is used for the treatment of a number of different illnesses, such as nosebleeds, pulled muscles, mumps (aka epidemic parotitis), arthritis, and vaginal bleeding.

Massage: A Great Way to Rest from the Rat Race

The third wellness feature I am going to talk about is the beloved by all Chinese massage. It is a form of treatment recommended in TCM for unblocking the patient's meridians, stimulate the circulation of blood and qi, loosen stiff joints and muscles, and strengthen the immune system.

Furthermore, it can be done to relieve symptoms without the need for complex diagnoses. It is commonly used for the treatment of back strain, pulled muscles, tendonitis, sciatica, rheumatism, arthritis, sprains, and other similar ailments. Another type of massage is the one called Tui na. In this type of massage, the medical practitioner presses and kneads various qi points on the patient's body. The patient does not need to undress; instead, they wear thin cotton clothes. They sit on a chair or lie on a massage couch while the practitioner presses on or manipulates the soft tissues of their body. Tui na means "push and grasp" in Chinese, so no, it is not meant to be relaxing or pampering but is a serious form of treatment for sports injuries and chronic pain in the joints or in the muscles. An interesting trivia is that Tui na is used to treat the members of the Chinese Olympic teams.

Getting Enlightened with the Fine Art of Qi Gong

We have already talked about qi but have only *mentioned* qi gong. Qi gong is a form of therapeutic exercise, an ancient Chinese style of physical training that combines preventive healthcare and therapy. Its purpose is to direct the qi to different parts of the body and it relies upon specific breathing techniques to do that. The term qi gong is literally translated as "the cultivation and deliberate control of a higher form of vital energy" – such an efficient language! Qi means the universal energy force flowing through everything and Gong means accomplishment through effort. Qi gong is the art of moving qi through the body using physical movements and mental concentration.

It has been practiced in China for centuries. Daoists have been practicing a form of qigong for around 4000 years to clarify and balance the mind. Along with Buddhists and Confucians, Daoists believe it can help attain enlightenment. Based on principles of Chinese medicine, the practice seeks to regulate Yin and Yang in the body and to maintain balance in the Meridians and in the Zang-Fu organs. Qi gong may be used preventatively, to promote and preserve health, or it may be practiced in response to specific disorders. Like other aspects of TCM, its greatest role is preventing illness by keeping the qi strong.

There are many different types of qi gong exercises and many new forms are being devised. The basic concept behind qi gong is the mindful harmonization of body, mind, and spirit in a focused manner. Hence, whether the qi gong requires movement or stillness meditation, the body is relaxed and the mind is focused on specific ideas or parts of the body. One of the most common areas of focus is below the navel and is known as the Tan Tian, which is thought to be a major energy center. According to the Chinese medicine principles, when the body and mind are harmonized through the practice of qi gong, the qi can be generated, blockages of qi can be released, and health can be boosted. Some qi gong styles involve movements that may be combined into graceful forms such as Tai Qi Quan or the Eight Pieces of Brocade, both of which have become a popular exercise for promoting health and reducing stress.

Other types of qi gong involve meditation and visualization exercises on a specific Zang Fu organ, Meridian, or even sounds and colors to achieve therapeutic effects in the body. Another type of qi gong involves massaging a specific part of the body while concentrating on balancing the qi in that area. There are many different qi gong exercises that may be performed standing, sitting, or lying down. Most qi gong traditions recommend that individuals practice once or twice a day for a general health prevention. Of course, patients with specific disorders who have been assigned qi gong exercises to correct a

"WELLNESS": A NEW WORD FOR ANCIENT IDEAS

pattern of disharmony should practice more frequently. The renowned Eastern discipline can be clearly seen even in the medical sector.

The practice of qigong is holistic; it can help the whole person become balanced and well by facilitating awareness and coordination. In China, it is used to help combat many health problems, like stress disorders, heart disease, diabetes and tumors while in the West, it is generally accepted as a safe, complementary exercise and relaxation practice. Calm, coordinated, rhythmic moves combined with deep breathing can still the mind benefiting the nervous system.

The idea of qi was broadly described in the *Yellow Emperor's Inner Cannon*. TCM practitioners actually believe that there are various kinds of qi. It is thought that various techniques, such as acupuncture, coin rubbing (Gua Sha) and fire cupping, can manipulate those various kinds of qi. Fire cupping was also practiced in the Western world and in Egypt long before Christ. The cupping technique was used in the Ancient West to manipulate the four humors of the human body. That rings a bell to the concept of manipulating the kinds of qi – again with the similarities, I know. However, whether East and West shared their medical knowledge this long ago has not been confirmed as of yet.

But what are those intriguingly sounding coin rubbing and fire cupping? Well, coin rubbing in Chinese is called Gua Sha, which literally translates to "to scrape away fever." If this sounds bizarre, the equivalent Vietnamese term translates to "scrape wind." Still weird? Anyway, it is an ancient technique used to cure a disease by making it leave the patient's body little by little as tiny, sand-particle-sized objects through the patient's skin. This method is also used in Indonesia.

As for fire cupping, or simply cupping, this is a form of traditional medicine found in more cultures. It involves placing glass, plastic, or bamboo cups on the patient's skin. Besides China, this same technique – though in a few varying forms – has been found in the traditional medicine of the Balkan countries, Iran, Mexico, Poland, Russia, and Vietnam – again with the alphabetical order, I know. In TCM, cupping constitutes a method of applying acupressure by creating a vacuum next to the patient's skin. The therapy is used to relieve what is called "stagnation" in TCM terms, and is used in the treatment of respiratory diseases, such as the common cold, pneumonia, and bronchitis. Cupping is also used to treat back, neck, shoulder, and other musculoskeletal pain.

Tai Chi: You Have Heard It; Do You Really Know It?

Another noteworthy form of therapeutic exercise of particular interest is tai chi, which is popular enough in many countries, mine included. It is a self-defense and calisthenics technique developed in Ancient China. It remains popular in China, where it is practiced daily and massively, often in the early morning in parks and other open spaces, while it gains more and more popularity outside its country of origin, as well. It is practiced in hospitals, community centers, colleges, sports clubs and elsewhere in many countries. In tai chi, the person moves through a series of 30 to 64 movements that require a relaxed body and correct rhythmic breathing. It is also worth mentioning that many Chinese practice tai chi as a form of preventive medicine.

Tai chi is not just a physical activity – it is a mind-body exercise that integrates slow, gentle movements, and controlled breathing. It also includes a variety of cognitive components, such as focused attention, imagery, and multi-tasking. Many health benefits have been documented by doctors and researchers in both China and in the Western world; those include improvements in balance, flexibility, stamina, blood pressure, general heart health, mental health, and symptoms associated with stroke, fibromyalgia, Parkinson's disease, and Alzheimer's disease – this is all pretty impressive, if you ask me. I should also mention that the more formal name of this technique is "tai chi chuan" which loosely translates to "supreme ultimate boxing" or "boundless fist."

Finally, there is a tai chi form called Yang Sheng Zhang and many Chinese people consider it to be as important as qigong to their overall health and fitness. In fact, many scholars state that qigong predates tai chi. Essentially, qigong is primarily focused on benefitting health and tai chi is a self-defense martial art. These two share many similar fluid movements with subtle differences and both practices are designed to promote the flow of qi or chi.

As expected, considering how much the Chinese love philosophy, tai chi also carries a philosophical story with it. So, in philosophical terms, it has a far wider meaning than the one its loose translations give. Its concept is used in various Chinese philosophical schools, usually to represent the contrast in opposing categories.

Diet

Earlier, dietary regulation was listed as one of TCM's basic elements. Actually, a person's diet is considered the first line of treatment in TCM. Other treating forms, such as acupuncture and herbal remedies that we studied, are used only after dietary changes have failed to cure the patient. Nowadays, diet is not an integral part of medicine anymore, though its benefits and influence are wholly recognized and accepted. In ancient times, however, before technology, diet changes constituted a true medical tool. Chinese medicine uses various foods to maintain the internal harmony of the body and keep it in a state of balance with the external environment. In order to give dietary advice, the Chinese physician has to take into account certain factors, which are the weather, the season, the geography of the area, and the patient's specific imbalances (not excluding emotional upsets) so that they can select foods that will counteract excesses or supply deficient elements. Basic preventive dietary care, for example, would recommend eating yin foods in the summer, which is a yang season. In the winter, by contrast, yang foods should be eaten to counteract the yin temperatures. In the case of illness, yin symptom patterns (fatigue, pale complexion, weak voice) would be treated with the consumption of yang foods, while yang symptoms (flushed face, loud voice, restlessness) would be treated with yin foods. More about the yin and yang philosophy is on the way, right after the dietary regulation part.

In Chinese medicine, food is also used as a form of therapy in combination with proper physical exercise and herbal preparations. One aspect of a balanced diet is maintaining a proper balance between activity and rest, as well as selecting the right foods for the given time of the year and other conditions. If a person does not get enough exercise, the body cannot transform food into qi and Vital Essence. On the contrary, if they are hyperactive, the body goes on to consume too much of its own substance. With respect to herbal preparations, the Chinese used tonics, taken as part of a meal before they began to use them as medicines. In Chinese cooking, herbs are used not just to flavor the food but also to give it specific medicinal qualities as well. For example, ginger might be added to a fish dish to counteract fever. Food and medical treatment are closely interrelated in TCM. A classical Chinese meal seeks to balance flavors and aromas and textures and colors in the different courses that are served, and at the same time, it aims to balance the energies provided for the body by the courses' varied ingredients.

Yin and Yang: A Can't-Be-With-You-Can't-Live-Without-You Story

And now, as promised, an analysis of the yin and yang theory is in order. We all know these two small words, we all love the black and white yin-yang symbol — many wear it around their neck as a necklace — and we all have a slight idea about what this duality represents. However, in this part of our Chinese chapter, we are going to dive real deep and we are not going to stop until we have found its very roots, its very beginnings in history, because it is the most fundamental concept of TCM.

So, let's start off by declaring pointedly that all things in the universe are either yin or yang. But — and this is the tricky part — nothing is ever all yin nor all yang; it is a balance between those two that is ever changing. Balance, symmetry, harmony, equilibrium: this is what yin and yang are all about. They are opposites and yet they are complementary. The yin-yang symbol is a representation of that Chinese philosophy and picturing it can help you understand it better. This symbol is a circle divided by a curved line into a black side (the yin) and a white one (the yang). The curve represents the constantly changing balance between Yin and Yang. Each side contains a small circle of the opposite color which symbolizes that there is some of Yin in Yang and some of Yang in Yin. To put it differently, yin exists in yang and yang exists in yin. They are not dependent/independent of each other; they *change into* each other. Well, without many examples, this is all just blabbering about. So, the day (yang) turns into night (yin) and winter (yin) turns into spring (yang).

By now, you may have guessed that, for TCM, illnesses are caused by an imbalance of yin and yang in our body. So, treating those illnesses would be, for TCM, restoring the yin-yang balance through one of the methods we studied earlier (or a combination between them). There are also eight parameters of disharmony that form a system in which illnesses are categorized. In TCM, illness is an internal lack of harmony, so only the knowledge of these eight parameters will allow the medical practitioner to perceive the location, severity, and nature of the disease process. This information will then be applied to the other diagnostic categories of qi, blood, and body organs, further narrowing and focusing the diagnosis.

Keep in mind that physical conditions are never fixed; instead, they are always subject to change. Inner processes evolve from a yin condition into a yang condition and vice versa. An exterior pattern can penetrate to the interior, a cold condition might turn to heat, and a disease of excess often becomes one of deficiency. And yes, in cases of more complex disharmonies, all eight patterns could occur simultaneously! For this reason, it is always a good idea to keep a Daoist attitude of flexibility while perceiving the movements of nature. Any diagnostic pattern is seen as simply a snapshot in time; an experienced practitioner should recognize this and always be prepared to adjust their diagnosis and treatment plan in a way that properly accommodates these changes.

Dualities in the Yin-Yang Theory

So, which are these eight parameters of such high importance? In fact, they are four dualities, seemingly opposed, one of them being the yin and yang duality. It is the most general of the four and it can be considered a summary of all them. Firstly, let's study the exterior/interior duality. The terms "external" and "internal" do not refer to where the pathogen comes from; they specify the location of the disease process in the patient's body. Our exterior is our skin and muscles while our interior is our bones and organs. In an external pattern, the pathogen fights with the body's defensive qi which circulates under the skin. In that case, symptoms include chills, fever, sensitivity to wind or cold, body aches, sore throat, nasal congestion, and a floating pulse. If the physician does not expel the cause of the malady, then the latter will penetrate the interior. In this case, symptoms are more organ-related, such as diarrhea, stomachache, intestinal cramps, lung pain, bladder pain, constipation, and changes in tongue color. In rarer cases, where the pathogen gets trapped between the exterior and the interior, the patient may exhibit such symptoms as alternating chills and fever, a bitter taste in the mouth, a wiry pulse, or a combination of those.

Secondly, let's study the excess and deficiency duality. A disease can be classified as an excess condition or a deficient one. Excess conditions occur when an external pernicious influence attacks the body and creates over-activity (for example, a high fever that is caused by a viral infection); a body function becomes overactive (for example, redness and swelling that are caused by an infection); or an obstruction of qi or blood causes pain. Acute conditions are usually conditions of excess. Deficient conditions arise because of an inherent weakness in the body or a weakness in the body's vital energy (the qi), blood, yin, or yang. Symptoms of deficiency include weak movement, pale face, pale tongue, and weak pulse. Finally, chronic conditions are usually conditions of deficiency. As a footnote, I would like to add that the term "pernicious" is the term that best corresponds to the Chinese one and we will meet it again in this chapter.

Thirdly, let's study the heat and cold duality. On one side, the possible causes of heat conditions are an external heat pernicious influence (for example, a virus that produces heat symptoms, such as a high fever), internal hyperactivity of yang functions (for example, drinking too much alcohol can cause a red face and headache), or

"WELLNESS": A NEW WORD FOR ANCIENT IDEAS

insufficient yin. The yin aspect of the body includes the lubricating and cooling systems. When these two systems are depleted, our body tends to overheat due to the deficiency of the yin. In general, heat signs include redness in the face, feeling hot, thirst, colored secretions (such as yellow mucus or dark urine or other discharges), constipation, burning sensations, irritability, red tongue body with a yellow coating, and a rapid pulse. On the other side, cold arises from external cold pernicious influences (for example, a virus that produces the cold symptoms of chills and rhinorrhea aka runny nose), an internal yang deficiency, or internal excess cold pathogenic factors. An internal yang deficiency produces such symptoms as feeling cold all the time, a low sex drive, and low energy. A patient with acute symptoms of loose stools and abdominal pains from eating too much ice cream, for example, likely has an internal excess cold condition. General signs of cold are a pale face, feelings of cold, lack of thirst, clear secretions (pale urine, clear mucus and other discharges), loose stools, muscle tightness, fatigue, pale tongue with a white coating, and a slow pulse.

And then, there's the yin and yang duality. Each internal organ has its yin and yang aspects which must be properly balanced. Heat, excess, and external conditions are yang conditions, while cold, deficiency, and internal conditions are yin conditions. For example, if heart yin is deficient, a person may experience insomnia, poor memory, and palpitations; if heart yang is depleted, poor circulation, pale face, purple lips, edema, and cold extremities may appear. When yin, with its cooling function, is low, heat signs occur. When yang, with its heating function, is low, cold signs occur. Restoring the optimum yin/yang balance in each internal organ is the most important "secret" of maintaining health and vitality in TCM.

▌ TCM Does Not Come Without Its Strengths and Particularities

Chinese medicine is very complex and intricate. Therefore, foreigners have to study for many years in order to grasp its unique concepts, which differ from Western medicine. It is indeed important to have a basic knowledge of TCM concepts to understand how Chinese medical practitioners do a diagnosis and how they treat an illness. This can be particularly tricky seeing that these concepts do not have a counterpart in Western medical practices.

TCM practitioners view the mind and body as the two parts of an energetic system that cannot be separated from one another or from the universe. Organs are not separate structures, but interconnected systems that need to work together in order to keep a body functioning well. TCM practitioners treat the patient and not the disease. The major difference that the patient will notice between the Eastern and the Western schools of thought is the much greater attention given in Eastern medicine to the tongue and the pulse. For example, TCM practitioners will evaluate the patient's tongue's form, color, and texture. When taking the patient's pulse, TCM therapists will auscultate three pressure points along each wrist, applying light pressure at first and heavy pressure afterwards, for a total of twelve different pulses on both wrists. Each pulse is thought to indicate the condition of one of the twelve vital human body organs.

Several of the advantages that TCM and other Eastern practices have to offer include a high level of patient compliance (often due to patients noticing improvements in their symptoms quickly), reduced stress levels, natural pain management, improved sleep, stronger immunity and decreased need for medications. Although some physicians and patients tend to be skeptical about the effectiveness of many TCM practices, research continues to show that complementary modalities can make a big difference in many patients' quality of life. Organs that are especially focused on during TCM treatments include the kidneys, heart, spleen, liver, lung, gallbladder, small intestine and large intestine. Depending on the specific type of treatment, the benefits of TCM therapies range considerably.

First and foremost, TCM reduces chronic pain and headaches. I put this benefit first, because it is of interest to most of the patients who use it. Two of the most popular TCM treatments for managing pain are acupuncture and acupressure. Acupuncture is most often embraced by patients who are looking to alleviate chronic headaches, pain due to arthritis, neck or back pain, plus many other symptoms related to injuries or stress. Studies have found that acupuncture, especially when combined with other TCM methods like tai chi and a healthy diet, can be valuable, non-pharmacological tools for patients suffering from frequent chronic tension headaches. Another research (done at Memorial Sloan Kettering) found that patients receiving acupuncture experienced less neck muscle aches and pain, osteoarthritis and chronic headaches compared to patients in the placebo control group. A research published in the *"American Journal of Chinese Medicine"* even showed that one month of acupressure treatment can be more effective in reducing chronic headaches than one month of taking muscle-relaxant medications.

Furthermore, a research conducted at Toronto Western Hospital found that tai chi contributes to chronic pain management in three major areas: adaptive exercise, mind-body interaction, and meditation. Trials examining the health benefits of tai chi have found that patients often experience improvements in five pain conditions, namely osteoarthritis, fibromyalgia, rheumatoid arthritis, low back pain, and headaches.

Second of all, TCM lowers inflammation and, in some cases, offers increased cancer protection. According to the *"Journal of Traditional & Complementary Medicine,"* TCM practices, including herbal treatments and the use of medicinal mushrooms, can have positive antioxidant, anti-inflammatory, anti-apoptotic, and autophagic regulatory functions. And you know how we love those anti-words when we suffer from any disease. This protects our body's cells, tissues and organs from long-term disease development. In fact, inflammation is the root of most diseases and, what's more, it is associated with the majority of common health issues, such as heart disease, diabetes, cancer, autoimmune disorders, and cognitive impairment.

TCM treatments can also help patients cut many harmful lifestyle habits that are related to inflammation, such as smoking, overeating, resisting chronic pain, chronic stress, and alcohol-induced liver damage. Overcoming chronic stress means overcoming poor sleep and hormonal imbalances. Some of the herbal treatments that have been found to directly help lower oxidative stress are reishi and cordyceps mushrooms, monascus adlay, monascus purpureus, amla, virgate wormwood concoction, green tea and its catechins, crataegi fructus, and the five stranguries powder.

Thirdly, TCM balances hormones and improves fertility. Research suggests that certain adaptogen Chinese herbal medicines contain antioxidants and anti-inflammatory compounds that can change the way that nerves transmit messages to the brain, this way improving various functions within the endocrine and central nervous systems. This helps improve the body's healing abilities in a natural way and also helps balance hormones – including cortisol, insulin, testosterone, and estrogen. Studies done by the Department of Food Science and Nutrition at Zhejiang University in China show that reishi mushroom supplementation can help lower symptoms of diabetes, fatigue and other hormonal imbalances, while improving fertility and reproductive health. By reducing the body's stress response, TCM therapies, such as acupuncture, tai chi and massage therapy, can also be beneficial for treating hormonal imbalances.

Even in the West, massage therapy has been recommended for diabetes for over a century now, and numerous studies have found that it can help with other hormone-related conditions by inducing relaxation, raising energy levels, helping people become more active, reducing emotional eating, and improving the quality of dietary habits and of sleep. A 2001 study published in the *Chinese Journal of Integrative Medicine* showed that acupuncture plays a positive role in hormonal balance and treating infertility. Acupuncture seems to work by modulating the central and peripheral nervous systems, the neuro-endocrine and endocrine systems, ovarian blood flow, and metabolism. It's also been shown to help improve uterine blood flow and decrease effects of depression, anxiety and stress on the menstrual cycle.

Fourthly, another important benefit of TCM is the improvement of liver health. Herbal medicine and nutrition are important aspects of TCM, since a poor diet can lead to liver damage – and the liver is one of the focal organs in Eastern medicine. The Traditional Chinese Medicine World Foundation explains that TCM views the liver as the organ responsible for the smooth flow of emotions, qi, and blood and the one most affected by excess stress or emotions. TCM, therefore, draws a link between liver damage and illnesses like obesity, fatigue, indigestion, emotional stress, trouble sleeping and many more.

A diet and herbal treatment plan that follows the TCM guidelines is very similar to following an alkaline diet, helping restore the body's proper pH and preventing deficiencies of key minerals. Stress reduction, exercise, sleeping proper amounts and many herbal medicines are used to treat liver problems. Acupressure massage is also used to stimulate the liver, improve blood flow and relieve tension caused by stress. Adaptogen herbs are commonly prescribed to improve liver function and prevent liver disease. Foods that can help improve detoxification and liver health, and prevent liver disease include raw and fresh vegetables (especially dark leafy greens), herbs and spices like garlic and ginger, healthy fats, and sweet potatoes. Alcohol, processed carbohydrates, sugary snacks or drinks, synthetic ingredients, fried foods, and refined oils or fats are all damaging to the liver and therefore usually reduced or eliminated when working with a TCM practitioner.

In the fifth place, it is recognized that TCM protects cognitive health. By way of reducing inflammation and oxidative stress, Chinese herbs can help protect brain health and memory. Cognitive disorders, including dementia and Alzheimer's disease, are linked to heightened inflammation, free radical damage, an inability to use glucose properly, vitamin deficiencies, stress, and environmental toxins. Therefore, an alkaline diet, herbal supplements, exercise, proper nutrition and reducing stress all help control the body's immune response and regulate hormones that protect the brain.

According to a 2007 report published in the *Journal of Clinical Interventions in Aging*, "There has been a long history of research and medical practice in dementia in China, during which the ancient Chinese people have formed a whole theory and accumulated abundant experience in the treatment of dementia." In recent decades, it has been shown through a growing number of clinical studies that certain herbal extracts (glycyrrhiza, atractylodes, rhubarb, ginseng, fructus lycii, polygala, angelica and safflower, among others) serve as expectorants and blood circulation promoters. Medicinal mushrooms have also been shown to help decrease the number of toxins or heavy metals that can accumulate within our body, thus promoting higher energy levels, better concentration, improved memory and better sleep quality (all important for a sharp mind and mood control). Coupled with other holistic treatments that promote well-being, they help prevent and treat many common age-related cognitive disorders.

In the sixth place of this long list, TCM helps lower the body's stress response. Acupressure is beneficial not only for liver health, but also for reducing stress. It is believed to stimulate a key point on the liver channel meridian, located at the top of the foot, that is related to emotional trauma and negative energy sources, such as resentment, bitterness, worry, anxiety and depression. Releasing these negative feelings can lead to reduced blood pressure, improved sleep, more energy, less muscle tension and more.

Acupuncture and tai chi can also be very helpful for managing stress. Tai chi is a type of qi gong exercise that is considered a mind and body practice, because it combines the principles of martial arts with controlled breathing and focused attention. The spiritual dimension of tai chi, focus on turning attention inward and quieting of the mind can help prevent cortisol levels from rising and improve one's overall sense of well-being. A study published in the *International Journal of Behavioral Medicine* found that, similar to yoga or meditation, tai chi is an effective natural stress reliever that can have positive effects in patients dealing with insomnia, anxiety or depression.

And last but not least, a seventh principal benefit of TCM is that it preserves muscle strength, flexibility and balance. Harvard Medical School reports that a regular tai chi practice can help address several core benefits of exercise: boosting muscle strength, maintaining flexibility, increasing and sustaining balance, and sometimes even providing an aerobic workout, which is important for the heart. Studies conducted by Harvard researchers have shown that 12 weeks of tai chi practice can help patients, especially those who are older or might have limited abilities, build a "healthy body, strong heart and sharp mind." Massage therapy and acupressure can also help improve

"WELLNESS": A NEW WORD FOR ANCIENT IDEAS

muscle recovery and prevent injuries. Deep tissue massaging helps bring blood flow to muscles and strained tissue, lowers the body's stress response (stress makes recovering from injuries tougher), decreases muscle tension, and might even help enhance athletic performance. Some massages rooted in TCM also utilize other mind-body practices like visualization, meditation and deep breathing to calm the nervous system.

THE MASTER OF HERBAL COMPOUNDS, AKA INDIA

For every stop that we will make during this seafaring journey in three continents, there is a term, a *historic* term, that can describe in itself the history of medicine in each country; its best part, that is. For China, I think we can all agree that it was the yin-yang balance. For India, that one term would be Ayurveda. If it sounds Greek to your ears (God, I hate this expression!), Ayurveda is the science of longevity. And if the people of India is not characterized by longevity, I do not know who is then.

The History of Ancient Indian Medicine

Indian medicine development started way back in 5000 BC (approximately, of course), when dentists in the Neolithic town of Mehrgahr, in the Indus River Valley (now in Pakistan), were drilling people's teeth to try and fix their cavities. About 1000 BC, medical practitioners in Northern India wrote the *Atharva Veda*, (also spelled as a single word) a medical textbook on disease treatments. Like the Egyptian medical texts written a little earlier, the *Atharva Veda* says that diseases are caused by bad spirits, so, in order to treat a given disease, you have to kill the spirits that caused it with poisons or spells. One example is the treatment of leprosy with a kind of lichen, which might have worked as an antibiotic. Another example is the treatment of snakebite by reciting certain charms.

"WELLNESS": A NEW WORD FOR ANCIENT IDEAS

The Atharva Veda includes mantras and verses on the subjects of wellness, physical and mental health. They are for treating a variety of ailments, charms for treating jaundice, fever, and some diseases, and also remedies made from medicinal herbs. However, it is not a plainly medical book, since it also contains other stuff about life, such as spells to gain a lover or a husband, prayers for peace et cetera. So, it is more of an ancient-social-folklore-wisdom-encyclopedia kind of thing, that did offer us useful medical information about that time.

Later on, the surgeon Sushruta, who may have lived about 500 BC, wrote a book, the *Sushruta-Samhita* (The Compendium of Sushruta), on his surgical methods. He described how to pull teeth, how to fix broken bones (bone fractures, officially) and intestinal blockages. His only anesthetics were wine and bhang (the natural intoxicant made from marijuana leaves and flowers), which he recommended to treat coughs and dysentery. A noteworthy fact is that he also described tuberculosis this early. About the same time, Indian people started using sand and charcoal filters to get clean water, which certainly saved many lives. But let's get back to our historical chronology and we will talk more extensively about this exemplary surgeon and his phenomenal body of work later on.

The Innovative Charaka and His Balance Theory

By 200 A.D., Indian medical practitioners had for the most part abandoned the ideas of bad spirits, and like Chinese and Greek doctors, they favored the somewhat less wrong idea of the three doshas (called Vata, Pitta, and Kapha) or humors. About this time, another notable doctor, Charaka, left a heritage that further helped promote health. Charaka recognized that prevention was the best cure for many diseases, so he recommended keeping one's humors in balance in order to retain one's state of wellbeing and stay healthy; this was a widely spread theory in ancient times. Notice how the notion of balance influenced physicians around the world. Charaka recognized three humors — bile, air, and phlegm (snot). According to him, if an individual's humors got out of balance, then they should take medicines to rebalance them. But Charaka also knew some specific medicines, such as citrons for the cure of scurvy (Vitamin C deficiency).

Indian doctors were respected so much that Indian traders got rich selling Indian medicines in Iran, East Africa, China, Sogdiana, and the Roman Empire. Charaka was the one to make the earliest Indian reference to smallpox and Indian doctors were the first to invent a way to inoculate people against that illness. Charaka was also the first physician to present the concepts of digestion, metabolism, and immunity and to describe the traits of a competent physician.

Another medical field of which Charaka knew the fundamentals was genetics. For instance, he knew the factors determining the sex of a child. According to him, a genetic defect in a child, like lameness or blindness was not due to any defect in the mother or the father, but in the ovum or the sperm of the parents which today is an accepted fact. Under the guidance of the ancient physician Atreya, another physician named Agnivesa had written an encyclopedic treatise in the 8th century BC. However, it was only when Charaka revised this treatise that it gained popularity; it came to be known as the *Charaka – Samhita*. For two millennia, it remained a standard work on the subject and it was translated into many foreign languages, including Arabic and Latin.

Nip/Tuck

The practice of surgery (Shastrakarma) first appeared in India around 800 BC. This should not come as a surprise, since surgery is one of the eight branches of Ayurveda, the Ancient Indian system of medicine. The earliest study on surgery is the Sushruta-Samhita (Sushruta's compendium). Acharya Sushruta was one of the first medical practitioners to study the anatomy of the human body. With the use of a dead body, he described it in detail in his compendium. He used to teach and practice around 600 BC and he has made significant contributions to various branches of medicine. His greatest contribution was probably the operation of rhinoplasty (plastic surgery in the nose). His detailed description is extremely meticulous and comprehensive. His wide knowledge of surgery is still relevant. The detailed steps of this operation, as recorded in the Sushruta-Samhita, are amazingly similar to the steps that are followed even in our days with such advanced plastic surgery methods and technological tools.

Together with the Charaka-Samhita and the medical parts of the Bower Manuscript, the Sushruta-Samhita is the foundation of Indian traditional system of medicine. In its 186 chapters, Sushruta has given descriptions of 1120 diseases, 700 medicinal plants, 64 preparations from mineral sources and 57 from animal sources. He has given precise descriptions of a number of methods, such as those of dissection, preserving cadavers, types of suturing and the material that was used for it, yantra-shastra (instruments), various operating procedures, bhagna (fractures and dislocations), kaumarbhritya (pediatrics), twaka vikara (skin diseases), Panchkarma, and many more (apart from his well-known work of plastic surgery).

Sushruta Samhita is considered as the landmark in the field of surgery and Acharya Sushruta is glorified as the "Father of Indian Surgery". He performed surgeries when no diagnostic facilities were available. Probably, it was his wide knowledge of basic science which made him such a versatile surgeon. His explanation of how to rebuild a patient's nose has given him the status of the first plastic surgeon. This was an important operation at the time, considering that amputation of the nose was a punishment for adultery in Ancient India. At the same time, the medical work Sushruta-Samhita is of great historical importance seeing that it includes historically unique chapters describing surgical practices, instruments, and procedures.

All in all, the most pioneering advances in the field of medicine were plastic surgery, dentistry, and the cataract operation. Indian medical tradition also goes back to the Vedic times, when the medical practitioners Ashwinikumars were given a divine status. The Vedic hymns of the migrant Aryan tribes are the earliest literary source on healing practices in India. These hymns provided us with unexpected insight into diseases prevalent during the period and also their perceived causes. The hymns in the Atharva Veda, which was largely composed after the Aryans were settled in the Indian subcontinent indicate that indigenous non-Aryan healing practices had influenced the Vedic healers. The

Sanskrit-speaking Vedic Aryan influence started to spread around that period and it was then when Buddhism, Jainism, and other new ascetic and philosophical movements arose. These movements promoted the idea of having a free spirit to question and wonder and experiment in all fields of knowledge, especially that of medicine. What fascinates me is that the importance of cultivating and showing compassion and having humanistic values is found in the very early Buddhist and Jaina texts. They were already recognized essential for health and wellbeing back then! – so, how can anyone say for certain when psychology was *truly* born?

Reaching the Core with Ayurveda

As I mentioned in the beginning, the key term for traditional Indian medicine is Ayurveda. Ayurveda is the indigenous medical system of that country, it has historical roots in the Indian subcontinent and it literally means "the science of living." Ayu means life and veda means knowledge. Unfortunately, the origins of this medical system are lost in the remote past and the body of knowledge that comes under the heading Ayurveda is ideas about diseases, diagnoses and cures, which have been accumulated over the ages. Many consider it to be one of the oldest healthcare systems in the world. The feature that distinguishes this system from other medical systems, such as Allopathy or Homeopathy, is that it is solely based on herbs and herbal compounds. On the other hand, what we do know is that the spirit of scientific enquiry influencing the intellectual world since the time of Buddha, something that led to the questioning of old beliefs, made tribal and wandering healers research more and learn more about medicine. Ascetic and yogic traditions, such as Buddhism and Jainism, and philosophical schools of thought, such as Samkhya, Visheshika, and Nyaya, were the elements that contributed to the formation of Ayurveda, which we can call a formal scientific healing system.

What makes Ayurveda a scientific healing system (and also art) is its disassociation from the magical aspect that tribal forms of healing normally have. Hence, the practitioner of Ayurveda could never degenerate to the level of a shaman or a witch-doctor. Hocus pocus and voodoo, which by the way are still widely prevalent in rural India, could not become a part of Ayurveda as it always retained a physical link between the disease and its cure.

The first Ayurvedic treatises begin with mythical accounts about how medical knowledge was transmitted from the Gods to sages at first, and then to human physicians. In particular, the Sushruta-Samhita narrates how Dhanvantari, the "greatest of the mighty celestials," incarnated himself as Divodasa — a mythical king — who then taught medicine to a group of competent physicians, including Sushruta.

Some scholars argue that Ayurveda originates from prehistoric times, and that some of its concepts have existed since the time of the Indus Valley Civilisation or even earlier than that. In any case, Ayurveda was significantly developed during the Vedic period and, later on, some of the non-Vedic traditions, such as Buddhism (centered upon the life and teachings of Gautama Buddha) and Jainism (centered upon the life and teachings of Mahavira), also developed medical concepts and practices that appear in the classical Ayurveda treatises. Ayurveda has eight canonical components, which are derived from classical Sanskrit literature. The two Samhitas we saw (one by Sushruta and one by Charaka) are written in Sanskrit and constitute some of the oldest known Ayurvedic texts.

The medical system of Ayurveda draws heavily from the doctrines developed in the Charaka-Samhita body of work. The main quality that Ayurveda has borrowed from Charaka is the aim to remove the cause of the disease and not just to cure the disease itself. In Ayurveda, there are no such things as instant relievers, pain killers or antibiotics. The herbs used in Ayurvedic remedies do not function against the body's metabolism; their effect is taking place gradually and, thus, there are minimum side-effects. The components of Ayurvedic medicines are largely based on organic matter. The absence of fast registering inorganic compounds which are at times corrosive, contributes to the absence of side-effects from Ayurvedic medicines.

This art — because then it was more of an art than a science — of healing was held in high esteem in Ancient India. It was elevated to a divine status and Dhanvantari, the most renowned practitioner of this art, was deified as the God of Medicine. Even ordinary practitioners of this art – the Ashwinikumars – were given a special divine status in mythology and folklore. Although very few ancient texts are available today, this method of healing was systematized early on. The fact that the term Veda was attached to this body of thought proves it.

Knowledge of this art was spread among sages, hermits and doctors who roamed from place to place. Those who practiced solely this art were called Vaidyas and they generally belonged to the Brahmin caste. Ayurvedic knowledge was passed down from generation to generation. But it is still surprising how the practitioners of this vocation did not obtain the status of a separate caste and how the vocation itself did not obtain the status of a distinct profession.

The wellbeing source that is humoral balance is emphasized, while the suppressing of natural urges is considered unhealthy, leading to illness, and this is when we get to the aforementioned "Three Doshas Theory". More precisely, according to Charaka, a body functions in accordance with the three doshas or humors it contains. The doshas are produced when the seven dhatus act upon the food one consumed. However, for the same given quantity of consumed food, each body produces doshas in different amounts, simply because every organism is different. Furthermore, illness is caused when the balance between the three doshas in a human body is disturbed.

The seven basic dhatus (tissues) I mentioned in the previous paragraph are the seven fundamental principles that support the basic structure and functioning of the human body. Namely, they are rasa dhatu (lymph), rakta dhatu (blood), mamsa dhatu (muscles), medha dhatu (fat), asthi dhatu (bone), majja dhatu (spinal and bone marrow), and shukra dhatu (semen). Furthermore, the Ayurvedic classics have categorized medicine in eight branches: internal medicine, anatomy and surgery, spirit medicine, pediatrics, science of rejuvenation (vitality), toxicology, eye, ear, nose, and throat diseases (what we call otorhinolaryngology today), and aphrodisiac. Ten arts that were necessary for the medicines preparation and application of an Ayurvedic physician were distillation, cooking, horticulture, metallurgy, sugar manufacture, pharmacy, analysis and separation of minerals, compounding of metals, alkalis preparation, and finally, operative skills, obviously.

Globalized and modernized practices derived from the traditions of Ayurveda constitute a type of complementary or alternative medicine. In the Western world, Ayurveda therapies and manifold practices have been integrated in general wellness applications and, partly, in medical use, as well. By the medieval period, Ayurveda practitioners had developed a variety of medicinal preparations and surgical procedures. Evidently, Ayurveda therapies have varied and evolved for more than two millennia; it is no static practice. These therapies are typically based on complex herbal compounds, while we also see the introduction of mineral and metal substances in treatises. Those substances were probably added to the mix under the influence of early Indian alchemy.

Moreover, ancient Ayurveda treatises taught several surgical techniques, including rhinoplasty, perineal lithotomy, the suturing of wounds, and the extraction of foreign objects. Even though lab experiments suggest it is possible that some substances in Ayurveda might be developed into effective treatments, there is no such evidence as of yet; Ayurvedic medicine is considered a pseudoscience. Other researchers regard it as a proto-science or as a trans-science system instead. For example, suppressing one's sneezing is thought to potentially cause pain in the shoulder. However, people are also cautious when it comes to staying within the limits of reasonable balance and measure – which is a school of thought found in Greece too, even in our days – when following nature's urges. For instance, people place emphasis on the moderation of food intake, sleep, and sexual intercourse.

Historically, Ayurveda has divided bodily substances into the five classical elements we have learnt by heart by now (earth, water, fire, air, and ether), just like the medicine in classical antiquity. These five subtle constituents of matter are known as the pancha-mahabhutas. Just do not ask me how the latter is pronounced. There are also twenty gunas (characteristics or qualities), which are considered to be inherent in all five substances. These are organized in ten pairs of opposites. That's right — here comes the list: heavy to light, hot to cold, oily (wet) to dry, dull to sharp (penetrating), static (stable) to mobile (spreading), soft to hard, smooth to rough, transparent (clear) to opaque (sticky), gross to subtle (expansive), and dense to liquid. Each pair of sensations is a continuum between opposites.

One of the views of Ayurveda is that the three doshas are in balance when each is equal to the others, while another view suggests that each human being possesses a unique combination of the doshas and that this combination defines the individual's temperament and characteristics. What is common in both cases is that each individual should modulate their behavior or environment in order to either increase or decrease the doshas and maintain the natural state of balance of their physiology. Ayurveda follows the concept of Dinacharya (daily routine), which says that natural functions, such as sleeping, waking, working, meditating, et cetera, are of great importance for health. Hygiene, including regular bathing, teeth cleaning, skin care, and eye washing, is also a key part of the Dinacharya concept.

Herbal Medicine

Which brings me to the most interesting (at least, for me) part of the Ayurveda medicine, that is the plants and substances used. For the plant-based treatments in Ayurveda, roots, leaves, fruits, tree barks, or seeds such as cardamom and cinnamon were used. Animal products used in Ayurveda medicine were milk, bones, and gallstones. In addition, fats were prescribed for both consumption and external use. The use of many minerals, such as sulfur, arsenic, lead, copper sulfate, and gold was also prescribed. In the 19th century, William Dymock and co-authors summarized a few hundreds of plant-derived medicines along with their uses, their microscopic structure, chemical composition, toxicology, as well as prevalent myths and stories about them.

We can see that Ancient Indian medicine had a great connection with medicinal plants. In fact, many of their medicines were made from

"WELLNESS": A NEW WORD FOR ANCIENT IDEAS

a combination of plants and minerals or even only plant extracts. Some of the commonest medicinal plants used in Ayurveda are believed to have been used since more ancient times. In alphabetical order, some of them are amla (Indian gooseberry), ashoka (Saraca asoca), ashwagandha (Withania somnifera), bael (Aegle marmelos), bhringraj (eclipta prostrata a.k.a. false daisy), brahmi (Bacopa monnieri), chitretta (Swertia Chirata), gritkumari (aloe), guggul (Commiphora wightii), neem (Azadirachta indica), peppermint, rakta chitrak, sandal wood, shatavari (Asparagus racemosus), and tulasi (ocimum tenuiflorum). Lots of spices, such as dal chini (cinnamomum cassia), elaichi (E. cardamomum), pepper and turmeric are also mentioned.

All the aforementioned medicinal plants and spices together with their beneficial effect on human healthcare could easily fill an entire book. Therefore, we are only going to study briefly a few of them. First and foremost, guggul, which means "protects from disease," is one of the most important herbs in the Ayurvedic tradition. Although it is very rarely used by itself, there is an entire class of medicines developed around its use. Guggul has very subtle and penetrating qualities and because of this is considered a *yogavahi*, meaning that it is often employed specifically to carry other substances deep into the tissues. Moreover, its combination with other herbs actually reveals its powerful detoxifying and rejuvenating qualities. Guggul can pacify all three doshas, though it is especially renowned for alleviating vata aggravations. In general, guggul has an affinity for all of the tissues in the body as well as the circulatory, digestive, nervous, and respiratory systems. It is also very scraping, which enables it to clear toxins from the tissues and channels while rejuvenating them. In fact, it is this scraping quality that gives guggul a number of its beneficial attributes. On a final note, let's see succinctly guggul's health benefits: it can purify the blood, help maintain normal cholesterol levels, kindle agni, promote healthy weight management, support comfortable movements of the joints, help engender a vibrant and healthy skin, and it can help women have a regular menstrual cycle. These benefits come in addition to the ones mentioned in the beginning.

Rakta chitrak is another powerful digestive and carminative herb in Ayurveda. It is mostly used for indigestion. Its botanical name is Plumbato zeylanica; in English, it is called (red) leadwort. Chitrak suppresses vata and pitta (2 of the 3 doshas). It works in reducing burning sensations due to its cold potency. It is a good anti-inflammatory and anti-diarrheal agent and it is also helpful in the adhesion of tissues and in fighting infections in the body. It can also work as expectorant and it assists in toning up the urinary tract. Finally, it provides strength to the body due to its sweet taste.

The beautiful ashoka tree was one of the most legendary and sacred trees in Ancient India. It holds an invaluable position in Hinduism, Buddhism, and Jainism. It is an evergreen tree that produces sweet-smelling flowers. It can be found in the Deccan plateau and in the Western Ghats of the Indian sub-continent, but thanks to its medicinal benefits, it is known worldwide. The barks, seeds and flowers of this tree help prepare capsules and tonics to fight various gynecological issues. It also reduces excessive and painful bleeding, leucorrhea and headache for women. Because of the chloroform and methanol properties, the bark is also used to cure bacterial and fungal infections. Thanks to the ketosterol its bark contains, it is one of the commonest household remedies for uterine disorders. Capsules and ointments prepared from the ashoka tree can be used as a natural supplement to treat irritations and burning sensations in the skin and complexion. When dried, its flowers are used to cure diabetes, while their extracted juice is used to cure dysentery. Medicine prepared from leaves, flowers and barks is used against diarrhea and purification of blood. Medicine prepared from the tree's extract can be used for the cure of piles and the bleeding caused due to that illness. Powder from its seeds cures kidney stones. The ground seed is also used as a memory enhancer and the paste of the seed is used for urine retention. Finally, even the ash prepared from that tree is beneficial; it cures rheumatoid arthritis and joint pain. And keep in mind that I even left out a few of its beneficial uses…

"WELLNESS": A NEW WORD FOR ANCIENT IDEAS

Looking for an Excuse to Have a Drink?

Therapeutic alcoholic beverages, which are called *Madya*, are used in Ayurveda, as well. They are said to adjust the three doshas by increasing Pitta and reducing Vatta and Kapha. Madya are categorized depending on the nature of the raw materials used and on the nature of the fermentation process. Their categories include: sugar-based, fruit-based, cereal-based, cereal- or fruit-based with herbals, vinegar-fermented, and tonic (either fresh or stored) wines. Ayurvedic texts describe Madya as non-viscous and fast-acting medicinal beverages, that enter the body and clean even the tiniest pores. Indicatively, prasanna cures flatulence, gastritis, piles, vomiting, and anorexia, while vibhitaka sura is good for general health, treats wounds, anemia, leprosy, and other skin diseases.

It is evident that Ayurveda, among other elements, incorporates a profile of alcoholic beverages with therapeutic properties. It is indicated that such alcoholic drinks, if consumed according to the prescribed procedure, in proper doses, at the proper time, along with wholesome food and according to the capacity of the individual, can produce effects like those of ambrosia in Ancient Greece. When used inappropriately, it acts like a poison and it can cause diseases. It is further important to apply the modern science in order to fully understand the traditional systems of human life; and the tradition of Ayurveda is so intricate that it requires a multifaceted approach of research for validation. The traditional beverages we talked about can certainly be investigated by modern scientific approaches to ascertain and/or find out more about their medicinal properties. Specifically, understanding of the microbes involved in the beverages' biomedical fermentation, the chemistry of fermentations, and associated biotransformation processes have to be studied in detail so as to validate the great and very much alive tradition of Ayurveda.

Purified opium is used in at least eight Ayurvedic preparations and is said to be able to balance out the Vatta and Kapha doshas as well as increase the Pitta dosha. It is prescribed for diarrhea and dysentery, for bolstering the sexual and muscular abilities, and for affecting the brain. Opium is not regarded as a sedative or a painkiller in Ayurvedic texts. It was first mentioned in the Sarngadhara Samhita, a pharmaceutical textbook. Opium was used in Western India as an ingredient of an aphrodisiac to delay male ejaculation. In the Bhaisajya Ratnavali, opium and camphor are used for acute gastroenteritis. In this medicine, the respiratory depressant action of opium is counteracted by the respiratory stimulant action of camphor. Opium's narcotic properties were recognized later and it started being used as an analgesic, too.

Oils to the Rescue!

In Ayurveda, oils are also widely used leading to wellness in a number of ways, including regular consumption, anointing, smearing, head massage, application to affected areas, and oil pulling. Liquids may also be poured on the patient's forehead; this technique is called shirodhara. Shirodhara can be one of the steps involved in Panchakarma. The name comes from the Sanskrit word for head (shiro) and flow (dhara). The liquids used in this technique depend on which illness is being treated. Among those liquids, milk, buttermilk, oil, coconut water or even plain water are included. Shirodhara has been used to treat numerous diseases or undesired situations, such as eye diseases, sinusitis, memory loss, greying of hair, insomnia, hearing impairments, allergic rhinitis, tinnitus, vertigo, neurological disorders, Meniere's disease, as well as certain types of skin diseases, like psoriasis. It is also used in a non-medicinal way at spas due to its relaxing properties. For those of you who might be a bit more interested, there are also specialized forms of shirodhara, such as ksheeradhara, thakradhara, taildhara, and jaladhara.

But the use of oil does not stop there either. In Ayurveda, both oil and tar can be used to stop the bleeding. In fact, bleeding caused by a trauma can be stopped with four different methods. These are ligation of the blood vessels (ligature), cauterization or cautery of a specific part of the body, use of preparations to facilitate blood clotting, and use of preparations to constrict the blood vessels (vasoconstriction).

Yoga and Meditation:
Two of Celebrities' Most-loved Practices

In the four shastras known as the Vedas, we also find the first references to yoga. The word yoga was first mentioned in the oldest sacred texts, the Rig Veda. The art of yoga, a relaxing and energizing technique of stretching the body and enhancing the spiritual awareness, has evolved through the centuries into a combination of techniques and treatments, now called yoga therapy. Restorative yoga therapy helps those who practice it loosen their joints, ease sore muscles, and tone internal organs through its many techniques. During a yoga therapy session, the energy lines (sen) and energy centers (marma points) of the human body are activated to produce vital energy (prana) which will alleviate symptoms of discomfort on every level — physical, mental or emotional. Some of the numerous negative conditions that yoga can relieve are: depression, insomnia, breathing difficulties, carpal tunnel syndrome, fibromyalgia, mourning, sciatica and muscle tension, autoimmune illnesses, nervousness, perfectionism, and many other ailments. Yoga therapy is also recommended for improving an individual's balance in order to prevent falls that might lead to broken bones. It has the ability to allow the body to achieve an optimal relaxed state. A body has to be fully relaxed to be able to receive the full benefits of prescript drugs; this is true for the benefits of treatments like chemotherapy as well.

Yoga's history has many places of obscurity and uncertainty due to its oral transmission of sacred texts and the secretive nature of its teachings. The early writings on yoga were transcribed on fragile palm leaves that were easily damaged, destroyed or lost. The development of yoga can be traced back to over 5,000 years ago. The beginnings of Yoga were developed by the Indus-Sarasvati civilization in Northern India. Yoga was slowly refined and developed by the Brahmans and Rishis (mystic seers) who documented their practices and beliefs in the Upanishads, a huge work containing over 200 scriptures. In Ancient India, the yoga gurus passed their knowledge to their disciples. In the pre-classical stage, yoga was a mishmash of various ideas, beliefs and techniques that often conflicted and contradicted each other. The Classical period is defined by Patanjali's Yoga-Sûtras, the first systematic presentation of yoga. The most renowned of the Yogic scriptures is the Bhagavad-Gîtâ, composed around 500 BC. Patanjali organized the practice of yoga into an "eight limbed path" containing the steps and stages towards obtaining Samadhi or enlightenment. A few centuries after Patanjali, yoga masters created a system of practices designed to rejuvenate the body and prolong life. They developed Tantra Yoga, with radical techniques to cleanse the body and mind to break the knots that bind us to our physical existence. This exploration of these physical-spiritual connections and body-centered practices led to the creation of what we primarily think of yoga in the West: Hatha Yoga.

According to a new American-Australian scientific research, yoga and meditation, can protect more effectively from memory loss. The study was effectuated by researchers of the UCLA and the Adelaide University and included 25 volunteers at the age of 55, who had all mentioned first signs of memory loss, such as forgetting names, faces, rendezvouses et cetera, before the study. These are all precursors of Alzheimer's Disease and dementia. The 25 volunteers were separated into two groups. The first group did yoga and meditation every day for twenty minutes, while the second solved crossword puzzles, played brain games on the computer and did other similar exercises to stimulate and refresh their memory. The test lasted for three months, after which both groups had seen improvement in remembering words, names etc. (verbal memory), but the first group, who had practiced yoga and meditation, showed greater improvement in remembering faces, places etc. (visuospatial memory). What is more, this first group was less possible to develop depression and stress, getting by more easily when confronted with various circumstances that may be stressful. The memory improvements coincided with altered neural activity, monitored using functional magnetic resonance imaging (fMRI) brain scans. Lastly, connectivity changes were seen in the brains of both groups, but only those of the yoga and meditation group were statistically significant. The study was published in the *Journal of Alzheimer's Disease*.

Other Medical Systems

There are also a few more formal systems of medicine, such as Unani, Rasashastra, and Siddha, that have been practiced in the Indian subcontinent. To start off, Unani is an Arab medical tradition that originates from the Greek Ionian medicine (the word Unani is actually an Arabic adaptation of the word Ionian). While it was being cultivated in India, Unani assimilated features of *materia medica* from the Ayurveda and other traditional sources. It is still popular and in practice in India and Pakistan.

Secondly, Rasashastra is an ancient tradition of healing that uses medicines incorporating metals, especially mercury and gold, purified using complex procedures. The tradition holds that, when associated with yogic and tantric practices, Rasa formulations can have outstanding results, like slowing down the process of ageing. Due to Rasashastra's effectiveness, certain Rasa medicines were incorporated into Ayurveda and Siddha, as well.

Now, the Siddha tradition is an ancient South Indian medical system that evolved mainly in the Tamil-speaking region of the subcontinent, where it continues to be very popular. It has integrated several elements of various sources (such as Ayurveda, Rasashastra, Yoga, and Tantra) and it uses alchemically prepared metals in combination with medicinal plants. The Siddha system has possibly been influenced after contacts with the Chinese and Arab medicines.

When talking about traditional and folk medical knowhow, we are not always referring to a complete formal medical system; sometimes, it is much simpler than that. That is, even before medical knowledge was codified into the canonical texts of Ayurveda, there was already an abundance of medical sources in the Indian subcontinent. Healing was obviously practiced by people from all social classes who lived and worked in intimate relation with their environment. Those... let's call them "healing methods" ranged from home remedies related to nutrition and treatment for usual ailments, to more sophisticated procedures, such as midwifery, bone setting and treatment of snake bites and mental disorders.

There were also specialists in bloodletting, experts in physical medical practices and others with profound knowledge of medicinal plants. Some healing practices were considered to be sacred and were associated with rituals that helped preserve them. It is interesting to see that in folk traditions there is considerable overlap between healing plants and that sacred plants and certain healing plants were revered.

Traditionally, even though folk healers came from all social classes, the Sanskrit-based Ayurvedic practice was addressed only to some parts of society. Although folk practitioners from the lower strata of society did not have that scholarly air, many who specialized in specific healing practices were highly esteemed. For example, it was not uncommon for scholarly Ashtavaidyas to look for help from folk healers in pediatric care, poison therapy or mental disorders.

To sum up this last part in one sentence, the original Ayurveda we talked about in the beginning has been enriched over the centuries through interactions and exchange with regional folk practices.

HEALING WITH AMPLE PROFESSIONALITY IN IRAN

Iran, officially the Islamic Republic of Iran, and partly Mesopotamia will be our third and final stop in the Asian continent before we get to the Mediterranean Sea, both in the north (Greece) and south of it (Egypt). Iran, which was called Persia at the time, used to be one of the intellectual centers of academic knowledge and a gathering place for renowned scientists from all civilizations of the ancient world. Iran was not only a cradle of civilization, but one of medicine as well. The history of medicine in Iran is as old and as rich as its remarkable civilization. The early rise and development of professional pharmacy in Islam was the result of three major occurrences: the great increase in the demand for drugs and their availability on the market, professional maturity, and the outgrowth of intellectual responsibility by qualified pharmacists. The practice and study of medicine in Iran has a long and prolific evolution.

The History of Persian (Ancient Iranian) Medicine: A Brief Presentation

The Academy of Jundishapur (3rd century AD) is one of the exemplary breeding grounds for the coming together of great scientists from all over the world. It was the most important medical Center of the ancient world (that is, Europe, the Mediterranean, and the Near East) and an outstanding institution for learning and studying in the fields of medicine, philosophy, theology, and science. Its medical students practiced on patients under the supervision of renowned medical scholars and physicians and they had to pass a special examination in order to obtain their professional practice license. Jundishapur scholars and graduates were appointed to important governmental positions. Centers like that permitted the successful maintenance of the scientists' predecessors' theories and teachings, greatly extending their scientific research throughout the centuries.

Beginning with Sumer in 3000 BC, sciences — including medicine, of course — have a long history in Middle East. We have to go back to the Ancient Mesopotamian period. There are many cuneiform scripts marked on clay tablets in cities as ancient as Uruk (2500 BC). Those hundreds of clay tablets that have medical content have survived from the library of Asshurbanipal at Nineveh (668 BC), an ancient Assyrian city of Upper Mesopotamia. The broad majority of those tablets are prescriptions, but there are a few series of tablets that have been labeled as treatises. One of the oldest and the largest collections (40 tablets) is the "Treatise of Medical Diagnosis and Prognosis." Although the oldest surviving copy of this treatise dates to around 1600 BC, the information contained in the text is an amalgamation of several centuries of Mesopotamian medical knowledge. It is a diagnostic treatise organized in head-to-toe order with separate subsections covering convulsive disorders, gynecology, and pediatrics.

Some of this information might sound like magic and sorcery to the non-specialist. However, the descriptions of diseases demonstrate accurate observation skills. Virtually all expected diseases are included; they are fully described and cover neurology, fevers, worms and flukes, venereal disease and skin lesions. These medicinal texts are rational to their core, and some of the treatments, such as excessive bleeding, are basically the same as modern treatments for the same conditions.

Just like it was believed in many other countries and civilizations in antiquity, in Mesopotamia and Iran too, diseases were thought to be caused by gods, demons, ghosts, preexisting evil spirits and the like. The rest of the stops of our journey are no exceptions, by the way. In this case, each sprit was believed to be responsible for one specific disease in one specific part of the body. Ancient Mesopotamian

"WELLNESS": A NEW WORD FOR ANCIENT IDEAS

mythology tells stories of diseases that were brought in this world by supernatural powers. One such figure was Lamashtu, the daughter of the Supreme God Anu, a horrifying demoness of disease and death. It was also recognized that various organs of the human body could simply malfunction, causing illness, or at least an ailment. Medicinal remedies were used to treat the symptoms of each disease, and are clearly distinguished from mixtures or plants used as offerings to such spirits.

At least four clay tablets have survived that describe a specific surgical procedure. Three of them are readable; one seems to describe a procedure in which the surgeon cuts into the chest of the patient in order to drain pus from the pleura. The other two surgical texts are part of a collection of tablets entitled "Prescriptions for Diseases of the Head." One of these texts mentions the knife of the surgeon scraping the skull of the patient. The final surgical tablet mentions the postoperative care that surgical wounds need. This tablet recommends applying a mixture consisting mainly of sesame oil, which acted as an antibacterial agent.

A very interesting and popular ceremony observed all over Iran was the cleaning of everyone's entire house for Nowruz (onset of the new Iranian year/spring equinox) and getting rid of all the uncleanness gathered during the whole year. What is even more interesting is that this tradition persists until today, and when people welcome the new year with a clean body, soul and neighborhood, they also start a fresh spring in their lives.

Medical Practitioner Types

There were two distinct types of professional medical practitioner in Ancient Iran. The first type of practitioner is called ashipu, who in older texts is identified as a sorcerer or a witch-doctor. One of the most important roles of the ashipu was to diagnose an ailment. In the case of internal diseases or in other equally difficult cases, the ashipu determined which god or demon was causing the sickness. The ashipu also attempted to determine if the disease was the result of some error or sin on the patient's part. He prescribed charms and spells that were designed to drive out the spirit causing the disease.

The ashipu could also refer the patient to a different type of healer called an asu. They were specialists in herbal remedies, and in texts they are frequently called "physicians" because they dealt with empirical medication applications. For example, in case of wounds the asu applied washing, bandaging, and plasters. The knowledge of the asu in making plasters is of particular interest. Many of the ancient plasters (a mixture of medicinal ingredients applied to a wound often held by a bandage) seem to have had some beneficial effect. For instance, to make some of the more complicated plasters, you needed to heat plant resin or animal fat with alkali. Once heated, this particular mixture produces some kind of soap that would help prevent bacterial infection. These two practitioner types often worked together and at times the same medical practitioner could function in both capacities.

There are also many drugs mentioned in those tablets (even though some of them are hard to identify). Surgeons often used metaphorical names for common drugs, such as "lion's fat" (much as we use the terms "tiger lily" for certain lilium species or "baby's breath" for certain gypsophila). Most of the drugs that have been identified were plant extracts, resins, or spices. Many of the plants incorporated into the asu medicinal repertoire have antibiotic properties, while several resins and many spices have some antiseptic value, and can cover the smell of a malodorous wound. Beyond these benefits, we should also keep in mind that both the pharmaceuticals used and the actions of the ancient physicians probably carried a strong placebo effect. Patients undoubtedly believed that the doctors were capable of healing them. Therefore, visiting the doctor could psychologically reinforce the notion of health and wellness.

Avesta

The Avesta (sometimes incorrectly called Zend-Avesta — I have to set the record straight once more) is the primary collection of religious texts of Zoroastrianism. It is a library actually, written in the otherwise

"WELLNESS": A NEW WORD FOR ANCIENT IDEAS

unrecorded Avestan (Ancient Iranian) language. In the Avesta, science and medicine rise above social class, ethnicity, nationality, race, gender, and religion. The Avesta texts also speak of consultation among Surgeons, Herbalists, and Psychiatrists, which indicates a form of medical association of the era. The first physician documented in Avesta texts was Vivangahan. Other notable physicians mentioned were Mani, Roozbeh, and Bozorgmehr.

The Vendidad (or Videvdat), one of the surviving texts of the Avesta, distinguishes three kinds of medicine: medicine by the knife (surgery), medicine by herbs, and medicine by divine words; and the best medicine was, according to the Vendidad, healing by divine words. It is actually the latest book of the Avesta, the scriptures of Zoroastrianism. The word Vendidad means "the law against demons." This body of work opens with mythological tales, or sacred stories. It also contains legal texts for both civil and religious situations, formulaic prayers for exorcism and ritual usages, and a sort of technical manual for priests conducting Zoroastrian rituals of invocation and purification. It ends once again with sacred stories; there is the story of Thrita, the first healer, who was given knowledge of surgery, herbal remedies, and sacred healing prayers by the Amesha Spenta Kshathra.

According to the Vendidad, in order to prove their proficiency, physicians had to cure three patients who were Divyasnan followers. At first glance, this recommendation may appear somewhat discriminant and based on human experimentation. But some authors have construed this to mean that, from the very start of their professional life, physicians were taught to remove the mental barriers and to treat adversaries as well as friends. Interestingly, a physician's fee for service was based on the patient's income. Similarly, the fee for treating a priest was (nothing more than) his pious blessing.

Moving on from the Avesta, in the periods following Zoroaster, the medical sciences continued to develop among Iranians, the main practitioners being Iranian Mobads (or Mobeds), who were Zoroastrian priests, and the Magi. The best teachers of medicine (and astrology, by the way) were the Iranian Magi. They are the only recorded designation of priests of all western Iranians during the Median,

Achaemenid, Parthian, and Sassanian periods. The Iranian Magi, who were renowned for their wisdom beyond the borders of Iran, and the Mobads were unsurpassed in their knowledge of medicine, philosophy, and plants. Fortunately, their knowledge was passed on to their students and kept its course down from one generation to the next. Unfortunately, the cruel invasions of the Macedonians, Arabs, Tatars, and Afghans destroyed many of the valuable writings and bodies of work of Iranian scientists, medical books being no exception.

The Achaemenid Empire, aka the First Persian Empire (550-330 BC), was an empire notable for incorporating various influences and civilizations and becoming the largest empire of ancient history. In the Achaemenid era, there were numerous physicians whose knowledge was used extensively by Greek scientists, as well as scientists from many other nations. The main bulk of medical knowledge in that age and even in the Median period before it and the periods after, was based on the Avestan sciences. During the Sassanian era, scientists from various countries, one of whom was Diogenes, studied different fields, including medicine, at the university in Jundishapur. The medical sciences stagnated in Iran following the Arab invasion. However, many Pahlavi scripts were translated into the Arabic language to save the books from Arab carnage and after some time, notable scientists were able to bring about a revival, and these sciences flourished once again; later on, they even exceeded past accomplishments.

We have to give credit for the establishment of hospitals and various training systems to Ancient Iran; there is no doubt about it. Jundishapur, in particular, is thought to have played a significant role in establishing for the very first time the institution of teaching hospitals (medical centers that provide clinical education and training to current and future health professionals). According to historical records in the Jundishapur International University, which was founded in 271 AD, had a double function; it methodically cured and treated diseases while medical students were trained simultaneously. Jundishapur was one of the three most important Sasanian education centers. The other two were Resaina and Ctesiphon. In the latter, the world's first medical conference was held, on the Sassanid King's order, in Ctesiphon

"WELLNESS": A NEW WORD FOR ANCIENT IDEAS

and it was attended by hundreds of mobads and physicians from Persia and other countries; a historical event that Ferdowsi verified in his epic Shahnameh. It is equally noteworthy that the Minister of Health (Dorostbod) was chosen from the physicians and the Minister of Education (Farhangbod) was an accomplished scholar of philosophy, logic, mathematics or psychology.

Let's Meet the Most Emblematic Personalities

Many scientists in the Islamic period made significant contributions to the world's medical knowledge, with only a few other people matching their achievements in this respect. Some of these great minds were Ibn-e Sina (known as Avicenna in the Western world), Muhammad ibn Zakariya al-Razi (known as Razi or Rhazes), Farabi and Omar Khayyam, among many others. These names shine in the history of medicine and will always be the among the pride of the people of Iran. These three scientists and physicians collected, studied, and systematically expanded the ancient Greek, Indian, and Persian medical knowledge and heritage, and they went on to make further medical discoveries. They were torchbearers whose discoveries tangibly improved human healthcare.

Farabi is known in the Arabic philosophical tradition as the "Second Master" after Aristotle, and Alfarabi (or Alpharabius) in the Latin West tradition. He is one of the major thinkers in the history of Islamic philosophy. He is a prolific author who adopted and commented upon Aristotle's logical corpus, while turning to Plato for his political philosophy. His metaphysics and psychology were a blend of both traditions which later generations adopted and adapted. As it was used back then, he wrote on a whole lot of topics. More specifically, he wrote — extensively — on logic, philosophy of language, metaphysics, natural philosophy, ethics, political philosophy, epistemology, and psychology. His treatises on psychology are called "Social Psychology" and "The Model City" and they were the first of their kind. He stated that an individual needs other individuals in order to attain perfection; that an individual cannot live isolated.

Psychology is a very important part of an individual's wellbeing. It has a definite effect on our body, our mind and our soul and it unavoidably affects any health problem one might come across. Psychology was also very developed in Ancient Iran. It was Al-Kindi who laid the foundation for explaining the problem of free will in a philosophical way. Al-Kindi noticed that the real action was not the result of intention or will and that the will of an individual is in fact a psychological power moved by their thoughts.

Omar Khayyam was one of the major mathematicians and astronomers of the medieval period. He was acknowledged as the author of the most important treatise on algebra before modern times. But, of course, that's not all. As most of the personalities we are studying here, he too had many different qualities. In fact, he was a Persian polymath, mathematician, philosopher, astronomer, physician, and poet, who wrote numerous treatises on mechanics, geography, mineralogy, astronomy, and music. He even developed an accurate solar calendar that was used for 800 years. Khayyam taught for decades the philosophy of Avicenna, especially in his home town, Nishapur, and continued to work in a variety of disciplines, including medicine, until the end of his life.

Avicenna (980 – 1037 AD) was a great and innovatively ingenious philosopher, among other things. Philosophers of the Islamic world used to conduct thought experiments even just for the joy of it, the most famous one being the so-called "flying man" thought experiment by none other than Avicenna. According to Avicenna, if a person is created by God in mid-air and is unable to see or touch anything, with no memories, then that person will be aware of their own existence. Avicenna does not even bother to argue; he just takes it as a given – and this is a fundamental thought in his philosophy. Any form of awareness of other things presupposes awareness of ourselves and the flying man thought experiment calls attention to our self-awareness. Avicenna concludes that we (our soul, our essence) are not identical with our bodies. This comes into conflict with Aristotle's theory that the soul is so closely associated with the body that it can only be considered as one of its aspects, which Aristotle called a "form." For Avicenna, the one

"WELLNESS": A NEW WORD FOR ANCIENT IDEAS

and only way to become aware of one's body is sense perception. Now, we may know that he was wrong, but his intelligence and ingenuity are nevertheless vastly recognized.

Ancient Iranian physicians believed that good health is the result of the 'right' measure of the elements of humor, and that sickness is the product of their excess or deficiency. Therefore, the medicine of the body consists of keeping the body in good health and re-establishing balance and the medicine of the soul involves curing the body and preserving it from sin. The Vendidad tells of three kinds of medicine practiced; medicine by the knife (surgery), medicine by herbs, and medicine by divine words, which according to the sacred text, is the best form of the three. A Mazdean physician-in-training was required to treat and cure three non-Mazdean patients before receiving permission to treat Mazdeans. In this way, physicians were taught to treat any and all patients, indiscriminately. Avestan scriptures did not restrict giving treatment to Mazdeans alone. The medical disciplines as delineated in the Avesta, were divided into five branches (Ordibehesht Yasht - Vendidad), as follows: 1) "Ashoo Pezeshk" (health sciences); 2) "Daad Pezeshk" (medical examination); 3) "Kard Pezeshk" (surgery); 4) "Gyaah Pezeshk" or "Orwah Pezeshk" (herbal medicine) 5) "Mantreh Pezeshk" (psychiatry, cure by prayers and divine words). The physicians were also classified into five corresponding categories, as you will see.

Let's examine briefly these five branches one by one. The first one (Ashoo Pezeshk) means health physician. It referred to both cleanliness of the body and the environment, as well as intrinsic health (that of the mind and the soul). In order to be able to cure others, the ashoo pezeshks must themselves be healthy in all the aforementioned ways. They were the physicians who oversaw the well-being of the city. They were responsible, among other things, for putting in quarantine those suffering from dangerous diseases, and for keeping the four divine elements (water, air, fire, and earth) free from pollution.

The second one (daad pezeshk) means medical examiner. These physicians were more involved with the science of medicine. Their job was similar to that of today's pathologists. Their duties included performing autopsies to find the root of diseases and finding a cure for the future. They examined the dead and, once they had ascertained the cause of death, they would issue the license for burial. If post-mortem examination was called for, they would do an autopsy. Mummification was also among their responsibilities, although this method – you could also call it a custom – was more prevalent in Ancient Egypt, which is the fourth stop in our journey.

The third branch (kard pezeshk) means surgeon. This appellation shows that those physicians performed surgery to treat their patients. In general, surgery is a very difficult and dangerous procedure, even today, but much more so in the past when it was not possible to anesthetize patients and medical instruments were rudimentary and only a few were available. So, as can be expected, many patients lost their lives during surgeries that were doomed to fail. This branch was not left out of the precious Vendidad works. As narrated in it, the physician must perform surgery several times and, only after passing the test, could they be active in this discipline. In the Iranian epic, Shahnameh, one birth by a "Rostamineh" operation (Caesarian section) is mentioned. The physician who did the surgery on Rostam's mother, Roodabeh, was Simorgh (Se'na in the Avesta), one of the famous physicians in ancient Iran. Simorgh was a Magi and he lived in the mountains, where his students went to receive scientific instructions from him. Because of his elevated residence on the top of the mountain, he was called Se'na-morgh. Lastly, it is worth mentioning that archaeological excavations in the city of Sookhteh in Sistan yielded some skulls that showed signs of surgery.

The fourth one (gyaah pezeshk) means herbalist. I believe it is only logical that the origin of herbal medicine not just in Ancient India but in any country has to go back to the development of agriculture and cultivation. How can you develop herb-based medicines and treatments if you have not learned your herbs to a sufficient degree, right? So, this part was not surprising. Now, one of the things that did surprise me a lot was finding out that the Iranian people was the first one to learn about the properties of herbs and to use plants in curing patients. I would bet my chips on another stop of our journey, but this branch of medical practice originated in Iran in ancient times and knowledge was spread

"WELLNESS": A NEW WORD FOR ANCIENT IDEAS

to other countries, such as India, China, Mesopotamia, Egypt, and many other places. After the passage of millennia, herbal medicine is still practiced in Iran and in other parts of the world, especially India and Pakistan, as herbs are considered among the most effective remedies.

Herbal medicine was also mentioned in the great Vendidad. It was used to fight numerous conditions and diseases, such as headaches, burns, fever, leprosy, snake bites, the evil eye, and even death. Many herbs were used in ancient Iran for instigating cures, such as mahuang (which was one of the strongest), wild rue, barsam and frankincense. Also, extracts from mint and Egyptian willow, as well as a distillation from forty-herbs, and others mentioned in the Vendidad were used as remedies. Some of those plants (including mahuang, wild rue, and barsam) also figured in certain religious rituals.

Finally, the fifth branch (mantreh pezeshk) means psychiatrist. The word "mantreh" meant inducer of behavior. It also referred to the divine and pure discourse that had the effect of calming and curing the patient. Mental disorder is a sickness involving the soul and the mind, and this condition cannot be cured with herbs and medications. Therefore, in those times, patients suffering from such difficulties were treated with indoctrination and verbal communication. Mantreh also included prayers that were recited to console the patient. When the human soul was greatly disturbed, the best cure was to recite the holy book (the Gathas of the Avesta), read poetry or listen to music.

Today, psychiatry is a pillar of the medical sciences and it is taught separately from other medical disciplines. According to Iranian custom and culture, mantreh destroyed all evil, filthiness, ugliness, and bad thoughts. God's names (101 names) were mantreh, the divine Gathas were mantreh, and so were Yasna, prayer, all the teachings of Zoroaster, as well as good thought, good discourse and good deed. Our forefathers believed and we too believe that when the soul and the mind are healthy and happy, so is the body. The reverse is also true, that whenever the soul and mind are weary and depressed, the body, no matter how physically strong, will become weak and wither away on a certain level. Psychiatry in ancient times involved reciting religious prayers and the Avesta, and reading the holy books of other religions and other nations. Through the centuries, the knowledge of medicine has been passed from Iran to other notable centers of the ancient world, such as Babel, the other four stops of this study (China, Egypt, Greece, and India), the Roman Empire, and now, all over Europe and the American continent.

Nipping & Tucking in Ancient Iran

The first cranial surgery dates back to the 3rd century BC. It was performed in Shahr-e Sukhteh (meaning Burnt City), in Southeastern Iran. The archaeological studies on the skull of a 13-year-old girl suffering from hydrocephaly indicated that she had undergone cranial surgery to remove a part of her skull bone and the girl lived for at least about 6 months after the surgery. Fortunately, several ancient documents still exist, from which the definitions and treatments of headaches in medieval Persia can be ascertained. These documents gave us detailed and precise clinical information on the different types of headaches. The physicians of the era listed various signs and symptoms, apparent causes, and hygienic and dietary rules for the prevention of headaches. Their writings are both accurate and vivid, and they provide long lists of substances used for the treatment of headaches. Many of the approaches of physicians in medieval Persia are accepted today; however, I think that even more of them could be of use to modern medicine.

There are several texts in the aforementioned Law Code of Hammurabi showing the liability of physicians who performed surgery. These laws state that a doctor was to be held responsible for surgical errors and failures. Since those laws only mention liability when it comes to using a knife, we can assume that physicians were not liable for any non-surgical mistakes or failed attempts to cure a disease. According to those laws, both the successful surgeon's compensation and the failed surgeon's liability were determined by the status of his patient. Therefore, if a surgeon operated and saved the life of a person of high rank, the patient was to pay a lot more as compared to saving the life of, say, a slave. However, if a person of high rank died as a result of a surgery, the surgeon risked having his hand cut off! Conversely, if a slave died, the surgeon only had to pay enough to replace that slave.

In the 10th century work of Shahnameh, Ferdowsi describes a Caesarean section performed on Rudaba (a Persian mythological female figure), during which a special wine agent was prepared by a Zoroastrian priest and used as an anesthetic to drive the patient unconscious for the operation. Although largely mythical in content, the passage illustrates working knowledge – as we would call it today – of anesthesia in Ancient Iran. Some traditional medicine forms are based on that description, with Unani and Greco-Arabic being the most famous ones. Obstetrics and gynecology in Ancient Iran were based upon the teachings of the Greek physician Hippocrates and the Roman physician Galen, and then they were developed by Razi and Avicenna into a separate and elaborate medical system.

The Four Humors

In Iran, we meet once again with the wellness theory of "the Four Humors." Only this time, a basic knowledge of this theory is simply used as a healing system in Ancient Iranian Medicine. This basic knowledge was developed and recorded by Avicenna (980 – 1037 AD) in his medical encyclopedic work called *The Canon of Medicine* (published circa 1025). In it, Avicenna also described numerous mental conditions, including hallucinations, insomnia, mania, stroke, nightmare, melancholia, dementia, epilepsy, paralysis, vertigo, and tremor. Recent animal experiments confirm the anticonvulsant potency of some of the compounds which were recommended by Medieval Iranian practitioners for the treatment of epilepsy.

Whereas Hippocrates is called the Father of Medicine, Avicenna has been called the Father of Modern Medicine. He is also called the Prince of Physicians. He was a Persian physician, scientist and philosopher who profoundly influenced medieval Islamic philosophy. He was particularly esteemed for his contributions in the fields of Aristotelian philosophy and medicine. Of his surviving works, over 100 address philosophical questions, while about 40 of them deal with medicine, including *The Canon of Medicine*, the *Book of the Cure* (a vast philosophical and scientific encyclopedia), the *Book of Salvation*, and the *Book of Healing*.

His influence over Europe's great medical schools extended well into the early modern period, with his body of work *The Canon of Medicine* becoming the preeminent source. Avicenna's penchant for categorizing becomes immediately evident in the *Canon of Medicine*, which is divided into five books. The first book contains four treatises, the first of which examines the four elements (earth, air, fire, and water) in light of Greek physician Galen of Pergamum's four humors (blood, phlegm, yellow bile, and black bile). The first treatise also includes anatomy. The second treatise examines etiology (cause) and symptoms, while the third covers hygiene issues, health and sickness, and death's inevitability. The fourth treatise is a therapeutic nosology (classification of disease) and a general overview of regimens and dietary treatments. Book II is a *Materia Medica*, Book III covers the diseases of human body parts and organs, Book IV examines diseases that are not specific to an organ (such as fevers and other systemic and humoral pathologies), and Book V presents "Compound Drugs" (e.g., theriacs, mithridates, electuaries, and cathartics). Books II and V each offer important compendia of about 760 simple and compound drugs that elaborate upon Galen's humoral pathology. It cannot get any more impressive than that.

Avicenna practiced Greek physician Hippocrates' treatment of spinal deformities with techniques of reduction, an approach that had been refined by Greek physician and surgeon Paul of Aegina. Those techniques involved the use of pressure and traction to straighten or otherwise correct bone and joint deformities, such as a curvature of the spine. Avicenna's suggestion of wine as a wound dressing was commonly employed in medieval Europe. Finally, he described a condition known as "Persian fire" (anthrax), correctly correlated the sweet taste of urine to diabetes, and described the guinea worm.

Avicenna's influence extends into modern medical practice. It was Avicenna's concept of *aproprietas* – a consistently effective remedy founded directly upon experience – that permitted the testing and confirmation of remedies within a context of rational causation. Avicenna, and to a lesser extent Rhazes, gave many prominent medieval healers a framework of medicine as an integral empirical science. Maybe this did not lead medieval physicians to construct a modern nosology or anything of that nature, but we should not underestimate the contributions of Avicenna, and the Greco-Arabic literature of which he was such a prominent part, to the construction of new modalities of healthcare that were fundamentally evidence-based.

The Resourceful Rhazes

Abu Bakr Muhammad ibn Zakariyya al-Razi (or simply Razi or Rhazes) was a Persian polymath, physician, alchemist, chemist, philosopher and an important figure in the history of medicine. A comprehensive thinker, the most free-thinking of the major philosophers of Islam, Rhazes was born in 854 in Rayy in northeastern Persia, where he was well trained in the Greek sciences. He made fundamental and enduring contributions to various scientific fields and is particularly remembered for numerous medical advances thanks to his observations and discoveries. His work in alchemy takes a new, more empirical and naturalistic approach than that of the Greeks. At an early age, he gained eminence as an expert in medicine and alchemy, leading to patients and students flocking to him from various countries around the world. He greatly profited from the Arabic translations of Greek medical and philosophical texts. A special feature of his medical system was that he greatly favored cure through correct and regulated food. This was combined with his emphasis on the influence of psychological factors on health. He tried proposed remedies first on animals to evaluate them.

An early proponent of experimental medicine, he became a successful doctor; he was appointed a court physician, and served as chief physician in the Baghdad and Rey Hospitals. He trained at the Baghdad *bimaristan* (literally 'home of the sick'). Like the European infirmaries, these were initially attached to religious establishments, in this case mosques, and medicine was taught in much the same way as religion. His main career was that of a physician and in that field, he earned great respect and wide acclaim. His medical works had an everlasting influence, like those of Ibn Sina. They helped generations of physicians in Muslim lands learn medicine; and, once they were translated into Latin, in Europe as well. He was among the first to use humourism to distinguish one contagious disease from another and has been described as the Father of Pediatrics and a pioneer of ophthalmology.

He is well known as the discoverer of alcohol and vitriol (sulfuric acid), as well. He was also an expert surgeon and the first to use opium as an anesthetic. Equally, he encouraged and pioneered chemotherapy in Islamic medicine and was the first in Islam to write a medical book for the general public, one of particular interest to the history of pharmacy. It consists of 36 chapters where Rhazes described diets and drugs that can be very easily prepared. Any person in their right mind can find the ingredients described and follow the instructions given. That book includes cures for illnesses such as headaches, colds, cough, melancholy, and diseases of the eye, ear, and stomach. Some of the ingredients mentioned are vinegar, sugar, poppies' opium, coriander water, rose extracts, pears, dried violet flowers, clover dodder, yellow arsenic, myrrh, saffron, and frankincense. In his book Manafi' al-Aghdhiyyah, Rhazes emphasizes specific matters and presents general regulations for healthy living. He talks about a variety of foods (bread, meat, fish, water, spices, fruits and vegetables, dairy products), their kinds, preparation methods, properties, and ways to use them therapeutically. He described the disadvantages of frequent consumption of wines leading to alcoholism and the numerous diseases the latter can cause.

To understand and appreciate Rhazes fully, one should look upon him as the product of his time and of the context in which he lived. Kitab al-Hawi was the largest medical encyclopedia of his era and he concluded it by giving his own remarks based on his experience and views. The author of about 200 books, he was constantly writing and his medical research was notably methodical. His magnum opus was the 'Great Medical Compendium' and other famous writings of his were those on Stones in the kidney and bladder. Rhazes advanced the medical field by making the distinction between the diseases of smallpox and measles. The latter's lack of dogmatism and its Hippocratic reliance on clinical observation typify Rhazes' medical methods. After having completed his medical encyclopedia, he also wrote a complementary book on the medicine of the soul, At-Tibb ar-Ruhani, which proves his concern for psychotherapy and psychology. His voluminous writings on medicine were universally admired. He classified diseases into three categories: the curable ones; the ones that can be cured; and the incurable ones. On the latter, he cited advanced cases of cancer and leprosy which, if not cured, the doctor should not take blame.

Philosophically, Rhazes was by his own admission a disciple of Socrates and Plato. He was noted for upholding the eternity of five primary principles (God, soul, time, matter, and space) and for a concept of pleasure that sees it as the return to a normal harmony following a serious deviation or disruption which is itself pain. Rhazes saw ethics as a kind of psychological medicine. The restoration of equilibrium following upon dislocation is the goal of spiritual or psychic healing, and preventing such disruptions is ethics. Rhazes' alchemy dismisses the idea of potions and dispenses with an appeal to magic, that is reliance on symbols as causes. He does not reject the idea of wonders in the sense of unexplained phenomena in nature. As he puts it: 'As long as the fear of death persists, one will incline away from reason and toward passion', which is an Epicurean argument. Finally, including unsuccessful cases in his notes, he showed that he valued progress and learning from such cases above presenting himself in a favorable light.

Finally, I would like to mention al-Tabari. He was a famous Persian doctor who lived in the early 800s AD and had Rhazes as his student. Al-Tabari wrote a huge medical encyclopedia listing all the different diseases that were known at the time and their treatments. He possibly influenced Rhazes to write his own medical encyclopedia later.

Remarkable Writings

One of the very first lawmakers in the history of civilization was the Babylonian king, Hammurabi (1728-1686 BC). The Code of Hammurabi (or Law Code of Hammurabi) was written in 1700 BC. It obviously included laws and regulations concerning a multitude of human daily affairs, but the ones which interest us in this study are the laws on medicine. For instance, law no.218 states: "If a physician performed a major operation on a seignior with bronze lancet and caused the seignior's death, or he opened up the eye-socket of a seignior and has destroyed the seignior's eye, they shall cut off his hand". Of course, there were many more laws and some that sound much more reasonable and human than the one mentioned. But I chose to bring that particular law up because I wanted to demonstrate just how much the generations of medical professionals have sacrificed to bring the science of medicine to where it is now. Physicians have lost their very lives – not just their jobs – when the result of treatment has been less than satisfactory. Even in the advanced societies physicians have lost court battles and good reputation for a poor outcome, even though they had no control over the course of events.

The most sacred texts of the Zoroastrian faith are the Gathas, seventeen hymns believed to have been composed by the aforementioned Zarathustra (or Zoroaster) himself. His teachings are general. According to him, laws have to change according to the time and the societal needs. However, religious laws are regarded as divine and immutable. He also speaks about attaining spiritual perfection (Haorvatat) and immortality of the soul (Amretat), and this is where there is an important relevance with our study. In the passages referring to science, the prophet is in search of knowledge and the truth and talks about spreading them. In the passages that are somewhat medical, we learn that the heart is considered to be the organ of thinking, while the mind is regarded as the center of thoughts. Even heaven and hell are nothing more than simply two states of mind. With his profoundly spiritual and spiritually profound words – I guess I do play often like that with words, as some friends have noticed, – Zoroaster, aside from a prophet and a spiritual leader, can be thought of as a soul healer or, as we would call that in contemporary terms, a psychotherapist.

Temples belonging to gods and goddesses of healing were also used for healthcare. Gula was one of the more significant gods of healing. The excavations of such temples show no signs that patients were housed in the temple during their treatment (as was the case with the later temples of Asclepius we will see in our journey to Ancient Greece). However, those temples were sites for the diagnosis of a sickness and contained vast libraries with many useful medical texts. The primary center for healthcare was the patient's home. The majority of healthcare was provided at the patient's own house, with the family acting as caregivers and helpers of the physician if need be. Apart from that, an important outdoors place for religious healing was near the rivers. It was believed that rivers had the power to take away evil substances and forces that were causing the sickness.

While many of the basic medical treatments, such as bandaging, began in Mesopotamia, other cultures developed such practices independently. In Mesopotamia, many of the ancient techniques became extinct after having survived for thousands of years. It was Egyptian medicine that seems to have had the most lasting influence on the later development of the medical sector; this happened indirectly, with the contribution of the Ancient Greeks.

Herbal Medicine

And once again, I am gladly going to talk about the most interesting part in every chapter, that is herbal plants and other substances used as remedies. The Avesta mentions several medicinal herbs including basil, chicory, sweet violet, and peppermint, while Bundahishn cites the names of thirty sacred medicinal plants. In the Vendidad, all the herbal plants that can remove sickness have been praised.

The Persians, who lived in an empire stretching from the Indus valley in the east to the Aegean Sea in the west with considerable variation in climate and vegetation, became familiar with a vast range of medicinal plants. In Ancient Iran (or Persia), various parts of a plant were used, such as the root, the stem, the scale, the leaves, and of course the fruit and the seeds. And they were used in many forms: either fresh or boiled or even burned on fire for incense and inhalation therapy. Their juice or oil was also extracted for rubbing on the skin and, finally, the ground seeds could be used in the form of granules or powder. What is more, due to their beneficial effects, medicinal plants were later consecrated and they entered liturgy. But we are not going to talk about that. I prefer to remain stricter and analyze only their beneficial role in people's health status.

A plant that is indigenous to the Iranian plateau is haoma (*ephedra vulgaris*). Haoma contains a large dose of ephedrine, which is effective in the treatment of cardiovascular and respiratory diseases. It is a small plant with beautiful yellow flowers. A juice made of it, called prahum, was found to be intoxicant and to cause drunkenness. Garlic was also used, whose therapeutic effects are well-known; it lowers cholesterol, reduces blood pressure and is also used to combat heart disease and treat infections. Wild rue was considered such an important healing agent that no tax should be imposed on it, according to Talmud (the ancient book of Hebrew). Wild rue was both a preventative and a remedy for poisoning. It was also a popular remedy for earache and was used to ease shaking fits of agues or joint pain.

Bangha, which was extracted from the seeds of Canabis Indica, has hallucinating effects and it was mixed with wine to deliver anesthesia. Frankincense was used for inhalation therapies. Aloeswood was useful for cardiac disease and for treating irregular heartbeat. There are also herbal plants that can treat the effects of certain toxins, because they have antitoxins. The following herbal plants are still prescribed actually: borage, sweet marjoram, fengreek, and chicory. Lastly, it is objectively worth mentioning — subjectively, not so much — that bull's urine has antibacterial effect, due to its high acidity. So, back then it was used as an antiseptic agent for the treatment of various infections and for the prevention of epidemics. Apparently, due to its effectiveness in preventing the dissemination of deadly contagious diseases, bull's urine received much attention. According to the Vendidad, it has a prominent place in sanitation and in the prevention of infections. In fact, bull's urine and fresh water were equally used for purification.

The Yasht Classification of Physicians

We talked about a collection of religious hymns, called the Avesta. After that, in Ancient Iran came the Yashts. In the Ardibehesht Yasht, there was a more advanced classification of physicians. In that Yasht, physicians were classified as follows: There was the Asho Baeshazo (sanitary physician), who prevents dissemination of contagious diseases, the Urvaro Baeshazo (herbal physician), or internist, who treats the patients with herbal medicines, the Karato Baeshazo (knife-physician), or surgeon, the Dato Baeshazo (law-physician), equivalent to a coroner or those who practice forensic medicine, and the Manthra Baeshazo (holy word-physician), who cured with holy words, an equivalent to today's psychiatrists. Manthra physician had a very prominent place among physicians.

The delivery of a newborn baby through abdominal operation worldwide is called Caesarian Section. It is named after Julius Caesar, who is believed to have been born through the abdominal route. This view has been contested much, because after his era, no woman survived that operation. However, there is evidence that Julius's mother lived long after giving birth to him. According to Shah Nameh, Rostam was too delivered by abdominal surgery long before Julius Caesar. Ferdowsi skillfully explains how Rostam's mother, Rubadeh, underwent the operation using wine as anesthetic. The historian Najmabadi has suggested that delivery of an infant through the abdominal route should be renamed "The Rostamian Operation." Well, if everything in this paragraph is true, then I certainly agree.

Exceptional Facts

And now, back to the Avesta. Didn't I tell you that each country's history of medicine has one term that somehow prevails? For India, that would be the Avesta, even if it's not an entirely medical term. The 21 books of Avesta were in effect the encyclopedia of the era's science consisting of medicine, astronomy, law, social science, philosophy, biology, general knowledge, and logic. Science and knowledge occupy a prominent place in the Zoroastrian doctrine.

The Farvadin Yasht reveres the fravashi (Avestan term for the Zoroastrian concept of a personal spirit of an individual) of Saena, a knowledgeable physician with hundreds of students, which denotes the existence of a medical school. It says that Saena Poure Ahumstute was a student of Zarathushtra who founded the school of Ekbatan. Plutarch (45-125 AD) writes that he studied in that university, that various topics of philosophy, astronomy, medicine, and geography were taught and that hundreds of students also studied there. The Vendidad names Thrita as the first skillful man in the art of healing wounds who was also acquainted with how to prevent them, as well as with how to repel diseases and fever. The Farvardin Yasht reveres the Fravashi of Thraetona for offering resistance to itches, fever, ague, and treating snakebites. Also, according to tradition, Yama was able to isolate the patients suffering from skin, bone and dental diseases. The second Ekbatan University was founded in the early establishment of the Median Empire (715 BC) by a group of Mobed-physicians. For the first time, the graduates had to obtain license in order to practice medicine.

The earlier-mentioned University of Jundishapur was an international educational institution founded in 250 AD, during the Sassanian era (224-641 AD) in the southwest of Iran. Medical science, anatomy, dentistry, astronomy, mathematics, philosophy, architecture, military commandership, craftsmanship, agriculture, and irrigation were taught there. The professors and the students came from all over the world. During the reign of Khosrow Anoushiravan (531-579 AD), seven Roman scientists, who had been exiled off their country by the Emperor Justinian, came to Iran. They were welcomed and well-received by Khosrow and were assigned to university posts. This was the glorious era of this scientific center. The scholars and graduates were later appointed to important governmental positions. For instance, the minister of health was usually chosen from the best physicians. Again, physicians had to obtain license to practice medicine. With the aim to

"WELLNESS": A NEW WORD FOR ANCIENT IDEAS

advance the medical science, Khosrow dispatched the famous Iranian physician, Borzoya (or Borzouyeh), to India. He brought medical and scientific books, herbal plants, and Indian doctors with him.

The first international medical conference was convened in 550 AD in Ctesiphon, under the patronage of Anoushiravan. Hundreds of physicians and Mobads, and physicians from other countries attended this conference. Ferdowsi has relocated this historical event in Shah Nameh. Due to the reputation of Iranian physicians, during the reign of Khosrow-Parviz (590-628 AD), a physician named Khordad-Barzin was invited to China and successfully treated the queen's daughter, who suffered from tachycardia. At the time, the sciences of pharmacology and alchemy in Iran were considered the most advanced in the world, and a total of 5,000 students studied in Jundishapur with 500 scholars teaching disciplines from various scientific fields. The library of the university consisted of eight floors and 259 halls containing an estimated 400,000 books.

SECOND PART OF THE JOURNEY: A MEDITERRANEAN CRUISE

Egypt and Greece may not belong to the same continent as do the three countries studied in the first chapter. But they do communicate through the Mediterranean Sea, so instead of giving this chapter the clumsy, kind of unfortunate title *Eurafrica*, I preferred the lovely Mediterranean Sea whose bordering countries can enjoy its world-famous and very beneficial diet. Besides, I could not leave the Mediterranean Sea out of a book talking about wellness. Historically, the Greeks have been a marine people with unprecedented love for the sea and shipping. Besides, we will see later in our study that doctors, scientists and other renowned personalities from both countries traveled around to collect as much information as possible and bring it back to their people and bring about a much-needed development in various sectors useful in everyday life, medicine being no exception.

In both these ancient civilizations, there was the belief that disease was a divine curse or a form of punishment for their sins. And in both cases, this way of thinking started to fade away gradually until it completely disappeared and pure logic prevailed. Medical theory and practice gained more and more ground. At first, people used to be based mostly on wishful thinking and lots and lots of prayer. Retrograde as it may seem, isn't it true that people still pray – often silently – when they are sick or even when they feel weak in some way? I believe so. Now that we are at it, I would like to add that, apart

"WELLNESS": A NEW WORD FOR ANCIENT IDEAS

from presenting many encyclopedic pieces of information, this study also offers you a great amount of food for thought and an organized platform for comparing the past with the present.

Traditional African medicine (TAM) is the medical system that features the most extensive use of indigenous herbalism. As expected, in TAM, the supernatural is believed to be the cause of illness. TAM has divination as a diagnostic tool and its treatment includes the ritualized use of a wide variety of plant- and animal-derived agents. Herbs are often used as part of a treatment in which physical characteristics, such as aroma, shape and color, and rituals, such as incantation, are more important than the herbs' pharmacological effects. Poisonous species are rarely used for healing, since it is not possible for them to be accurately measured.

Back to our two beloved and world-changing ancient civilizations. Not all Ancient Greek and Egyptian medicine was based on wishful thinking; much of it was the result of experimentation and observation, and physical means supplemented the magical ones. Apart from spiritual healing and herbal medicine, Ancient Egyptians practiced massage and made extensive use of therapeutic herbs and foods, but surgery was only rarely part of their treatments. According to Herodotus, who traveled several times in Egypt, there was a high degree of specialization among physicians.

The Egyptians were advanced medical practitioners for their time. They were masters of human anatomy and healing mostly due to the extensive mummification ceremonies. This involved removing most of the internal organs, including the brain, lungs, pancreas, liver, spleen, heart and intestine. To some extent, they had a basic knowledge of organ functions within the human body. Their great knowledge of anatomy, as well as (mostly in the later dynasties) the crossover of knowledge between the Greek and other cultures led to an extensive knowledge of the functioning of the organs, and branched into many other medical practices.

Herodotus and Pliny were among the Greek scholars, who benefitted from this crossover and further contributed to the ancient (and modern) medical progress, starting then and there and, unbeknownst to them, reaching eternity by discovering and recording things we still use and value in our days. Ancient Egyptians were as equally familiar with pharmacy as they were with medicine. According to historical records, they used to recite certain incantations while preparing or administering medications. So, the former were included in the medical and pharmaceutical professions. They were also familiar with drug preparation from plants and herbs, such as cumin, fennel, caraway, aloe, safflower, pomegranates, castor and linseed oil. Other drugs were made of mineral substances such as copper salts, plain salt and lead. Several other products, such as eggs, liver, hairs, milk, animal horns and fat, honey, and wax, were also used in drug preparation.

The Ancient Greeks, some 1000 years before the birth of Jesus Christ, recognized the importance of physicians and their art. As related in the works of Homer, injured warriors were treated by physicians. They continued to develop the art of medicine and made many advances, although they were not as skilled as the Ancient Egyptians, whom even Homer recognized as the greatest healers in the world.

Whilst they imported much of their medical knowledge from the Egyptians, they did develop some skills of their own and certainly influenced the course of the Western history of medicine. The pivotal moment in the return of Greek medical knowledge to Europe was the arrival of Constantine of Africa at the Southern Italian port of Salerno around 1075. Little is known for certain about him. He was born a Muslim, probably at Carthage, North Africa. Earlier in his life he may have travelled to India and Ethiopia, but certainly visited Damascus, possibly studying at the *bimaristan* there. He later returned to Carthage, but was thought to be a wizard and was forced to flee for his life, which probably explains his arrival in Salerno.

The Ancient Greeks tended to believe that most ailments could be healed by prayers to the God of Medicine, Asclepius, and the great temples, known as Asclepeions, were where many people went to seek healing, making sacrifices and praying to Asclepius in return for having their ailments healed. However, this all changed when Hippocrates, one of the most famous and one of the most prolific out of all physicians, came. His around-the-world famous oath is still used by all doctors – no

"WELLNESS": A NEW WORD FOR ANCIENT IDEAS

matter their field of specialization – today, as they pledge to 'Do No Harm,' among other things, of course. Hippocrates's most distinct contribution to the history of medicine was the separation of medicine from the divine element. He believed that checking symptoms, giving diagnoses and administering treatment should be separated from the rituals of the priests, although most Greeks were happy to place their bets on a combination of the two.

Greek doctors, influenced by the Hippocratic thought, would study the case history of patients, asking questions and attempting to find out as much as possible from the patient before reaching a final diagnosis. This two-way interaction between the patient and the doctor actually became a fundamental practice in the field of medicine that is still being used by modern-day medical practitioners.

Furthermore, the Ancient Greeks believed that there were four humors making up the human body, and an imbalance within these humors would lead to sickness (both mental and physical illnesses and ailments). The balance of these humors would be affected by diet, location, age, climate and a range of other factors, and Ancient Greek medicine was based upon restoring the balance. I am not going to name the four humors and the significance of each one right now; these are all explicitly studied in the chapter about Ancient Greece. Many of the Greek herbal remedies and medicines were based around restoring the balance of the four humors, and this belief continued prevailing in the European thought well into the Middle Ages.

The Greeks were also surgeons and some of the equipment they used is recognizable to this day. Some of their tools included forceps, scalpels, tooth-extraction forceps and catheters, and there were even syringes for drawing pus from wounds. One instrument, the spoon of Diocles, was used by the surgeon Kritoboulos, to remove the injured eye of Phillip of Macedon without undue scarring. Finally, the Greeks knew how to splint and treat bone fractures, as well as add compresses to prevent infections.

So, in conclusion, Ancient Egyptians and Ancient Greeks laid down the roots of the modern history of medicine, understanding the value of cleanliness, medicines and the finer art of various surgical procedures. Their knowledge was then passed down to the Romans, who preserved their predecessors' medical skills and refined them. Anyone interested in a medical career should seriously consider studying Latin or Greek – ideally both. The Greeks developed the first specialized medical vocabulary in the Western world. It was a Later, the Romans inherited it and translated it into Latin, setting the stage for their introduction into the modern Romance languages and the English language. The revival of classical learning in the Renaissance further contributed to the growth of a consistent medical vocabulary in Europe. To this day, the naming of new scientific words involves the formation of Greek and Latin compounds that are imported into all modern languages of scientific relevance (the International Scientific Vocabulary).

TREATING WITH A PINCH OF ARTISTRY IN EGYPT

A Short History of Ancient Egyptian Medicine

The Ancient Egyptian civilization was the first great civilization on Earth. It was not only the majestic pyramids and tombs we all know and admire, but it involved all aspects of human life. In actuality, it is in Egypt that we see the onset of what we today call medical care. What is more, most of the complementary medicine modalities were originated from the Ancient Egyptians. One of these modalities is herbal medicine, which is my favorite part, because it also involves nature that I love dearly; we are going to study that part later on in the study. Health and wellbeing was one of the most cared arts by the pharaohs. And, no, I am not calling it "art" by mistake; again, I will explain later what I mean exactly.

Ancient Egypt (3300-525 BC) is another country where disease was thought to be a divine intervention, simply because there was no other way to explain it. And the diseases' causes were definitely mysterious, so Egyptians ended up believing that gods and demons and evil spirits (such as Wehedu) with their poisons played a key role in making someone suffer through a disease. They thought that gods were the creators and controllers of life. They believed conception was carried out by the mighty god Thoth, while Bes, another strong goddess, decided whether childbirth would go smoothly or would be painstaking and exhausting. As a result of those beliefs, both the physicians and magicians participated in the field of medical care.

From a holistic point of view, they perceived health and sickness as an unceasing fight between good and evil.

At the time, physicians believed that spirits blocked certain channels in the human body, affecting consequently the way the body normally functioned. Therefore, their research at first involved trying to find ways to unblock the blocked channels; with the use of laxatives, for instance. Cleansing the body was the way to rid the patient of the superhuman influence. Numerous discovered papyrus documents are from the era between 1900 and 1500 BC. It is from those documents that we have learnt that the Ancient Egyptians still believed at that time that supernatural forces caused diseases. Actually, the knowledge we have about Ancient Egyptian medicine comes almost in its entirety from papyri. When discovered, many of those papyrus documents were very well-preserved — considering their age, that is — thanks to the very dry climate of Egypt.

Actually, this thing about channels is a true and pretty complete theory. It was conceived while observing farmers who dug irrigation channels to water their crops. They believed that, much like in irrigation, the body had channels that provided it with routes for good health. The heart was believed to be the center of 46 channels. Consider them as any kind of tube. And we have to admit that, to a certain extent, they had it right; our veins, our arteries, and even our intestines can be perceived as types of tubes. Ancient Egyptians did not come to realize that each of these channels has a different function, but on the other hand, it was the channel theory that allowed medicine to move from entirely spiritual cures for diseases and ailments towards more practical ones. According to many medical historians, this change was a major turning point, a real breakthrough in the history of medicine.

In the beginning, preventive methods included prayers and various kinds of magic, in addition to all their world-famous heavy amulet-wearing. There were numerous incantations and prayers to the gods — above all to Sekhmet, the goddess of healing — and also curses and threats. All those were accompanied by the injection of medicines into the various bodily orifices and were hoped to prove effective. On a side note, said medicines had both a bad taste and a bad smell.

"WELLNESS": A NEW WORD FOR ANCIENT IDEAS

The wab Sekhmet (priest-physician) had a number of important functions. First of all, to discover the nature of the particular entity possessing the person and then attack, drive it out, or otherwise destroy it. This was done by some powerful magic for which rituals, spells, incantations, talismans and amulets were used. Sekhmet priests seem also to have been involved in the prevention of plagues, inspection of sacrificial animals and even veterinary medicine. Other types of healers like the sunu and the sau seem to have had recourse to the same methods and scriptures as the wab.

But, do not be fooled by all that. If I had to be sick in those ancient times, the place I would choose would probably be Egypt. It is not that my chances of survival in Ancient Egypt would be that significantly higher than those in other countries — after all, there was no technology anywhere — but at least I would have the satisfaction of being in good hands and being treated by doctors whose art was renowned all over the ancient world. Yes, we are talking about healing and treating as a form of art again. Before being able to be called a science, medicine was and should be considered an art. Viewing developed medicine as an art in certain ancient countries helps distinguish those countries among others where health care was practiced with somewhat primitive methods.

Egyptian doctors gradually started to use combinations of natural remedies, together with prayer, and through a process of trial and error and some basic science of course, medical care was seen as a profession. They were trained and good at practical first aid. They could also fix successfully broken bones and dislocated joints. They had bandages of very good quality and in them they would wrap certain plant products, such as willow leaves, for the treatment of inflammation. Rulers in Ancient Egypt sponsored physicians that were specialists in specific diseases. Imhotep was the first medical doctor known by name. An Egyptian who lived around 2650 BC, he was an adviser to King Zoser at a time when Egyptians were making progress in medicine. Among his contributions to medicine was a textbook on the treatment of wounds, broken bones, and even tumors.

Unlike the illnesses and their causes which were unknown and mysterious, the injuries caused by accidents or fighting were taken care of by the sunu. Other types of wounds, such as scorpion stings and snake bites, were dealt with by the Kherep Serqet (the exorcist of Serqet), who knew the appropriate spells and remedies. The significant role that food played was also recognized on a sufficient level. Our natural craving for diversity combined with well-irrigated soil resulted in a diet that was astonishingly balanced. Ancient Egyptians received carbohydrates from cereals, vitamins from fruit and vegetables, and proteins mostly from fish. They also consumed legumes, seeds, oil, milk and dairy products occasionally.

Suffering from Frequent Diseases

Much like we do today, Ancient Egyptians too suffered from all the everyday ailments, diseases and simple disorders, such as stomachaches, headaches, common colds, diarrhea, intestinal issues, bowel troubles and other lovely ailments. They had simple remedies made from natural ingredients, like grains and seeds, honey, oil, staghorn, and water, for such conditions. The common cold probably plagued the Ancient Egyptians much like it still annoys us today. Of course, today, we can take a couple of pills for rhinorrhea and diarrhea while back then the remedy for common cold was the milk of a mother who has given birth to a boy – in Greek, there is a compound word that describes that; it would correspond to a term like "boymother." But, apart from that special motherly milk, they also had a tried and true spell to go with it, which is written in the precious Ebers Papyrus.

Insect-borne diseases, such as malaria and trachoma, an eye disease, were endemic in Ancient Egypt. Plagues would spread along the trade routes which were of vital importance to the economy of the country. Moreover, a number of *yadet renpet* epidemics mentioned in some papyri are thought to have been outbreaks of bubonic plagues. Mosquitoes also spread filarial worms which caused elephantiasis, a disfiguring disease. This did not appear very frequently; it caused, however, tremendous suffering to the patients.

"WELLNESS": A NEW WORD FOR ANCIENT IDEAS

Infectious diseases were pretty uncontrollable in the relatively densely populated Nile valley. Practically the entire population there lived within a narrow strip of land along the river, which at times was only a few hundred meters wide, and the diseases' incidence depended to some degree on the seasons. Diseases such as smallpox, diarrhea, dysentery, typhoid, jaundice, and relapsing fever were responsible for many deaths, above all during the spring and summer. The ubiquity of water during the floods brought with it a whole new set of ailments, with malaria being probably the central one. Said diseases were the main cause for mortality in autumn. On the other hand, the cooler weather of autumn and winter seems to have favored the outbreak of respiratory illnesses. Instances of diseases which are rare today, such as osteopetrosis, were also found.

Naturally, there were also animal-specific diseases. Trichinae afflicted the pigs, parasitic worms and tuberculosis the cattle and they were occasionally passed on to the human population. In fact, human tuberculosis was widespread; leprosy, on the other hand, caused by bacteria similar to the *tubercle bacillus*, is badly documented and was apparently relatively rare, possibly because of an immunity tuberculosis sufferers acquired. According to some researchers, leprosy originated in Egypt and spread to the Levant and Europe along the migration and trade routes, while according to others, there is no proof of its existence in ancient times. The daily hard work, which was often repetitive, caused great harm to the bones and joints of the laborers after only a few years of doing it. Those who survived to live a longer life were victims of the same infirmities that still plague the elderly, such as cardio-vascular diseases, arthritis, from which Ramses II suffered, and probably dementia. Silicosis of the lungs, which is the result of breathing in airborne sand particles, was a frequent cause of death. Pneumonia was one, too. Lastly, the various kinds of malignant tumors were almost as frequent then as they are nowadays in comparable age and gender groups.

Congenital diseases were not uncommon and often brought about early death as the numerous burials of infants show. Their causes may have been environmental, nutritional or social. Inbreeding, not infrequent among the royals, was probably also not rare among the common people largely bound to the soil: the occurrence of a sixth finger or toe in mummies, interpreted by some as the result of inbreeding, has been noted a number of times. Open wounds were often treated with honey, but sepsis was one of the commonest causes of death. When lockjaw set in due to a tetanus infection, physicians knew they were powerless against this new affliction.

Concerning eye infections, they are a common ailment in the African continent. In Ancient Egypt, though, they were (at least partly) prevented by the application of bactericidal eye paint. The ingredients of some of those remedies may not have been as difficult to come by in a civilization, where the brain of the dead was removed in little bits from the skull during mummification and discarded, as it would be in a modern western country.

Little is known about pregnancy and childbirth in Ancient Egypt, and on the basis of a few literary hints, one surmises that, unless there was some extraordinary problem, physicians were not involved. There was a store of knowledge concerning women, as is reflected in the Kahun Gynecological Papyrus, the Greater Berlin Papyrus and others, which dealt with urinary problems, pains in the abdomen, legs and genitals, fertility and conception.

Surgery and Circumcision

Basic surgery, meaning procedures close to the surface of the skin (or on the skin) was a common and well-learnt skill; they knew how to stitch wounds effectively. They did not, however, perform surgery deep inside the human body. They had no effective anesthetics – only antiseptics. Performing surgery deep inside a human body would have been impossible. Circumcision of baby boys was also a common practice. Egyptian surgeons already had an impressive array of instruments in their disposition, such as pincers, forceps, spoons, bone saws, scalpels, containers with burning incense, retractors, suction cups, scales, hooks, lances, knives, chisels, and dental tools. All these instruments were found illustrating Ancient Egyptian inscriptions.

"WELLNESS": A NEW WORD FOR ANCIENT IDEAS

There were also prosthetic parts, but their role was not medical because they were not as functional as today's technology can make them. They were only used for decorative purposes in funerals. Egyptians wanted to make the departed look good and, if needed, they added prosthetic parts in the coffin of departed handicapped individuals. So, prostheses were of a cosmetic character, such as an artificial toe made of cartonnage found in the British Museum, or were added as a preparation for afterlife, such as a forearm on a mummy found in Arlington Museum and an artificial penis and feet on another mummy in the Manchester Museum. Cartonnage is a type of material used widely in Ancient Egyptian funerary masks from the First Intermediate Period to the Roman era. A wooden big toe prosthesis has also been found which might have improved the walking capabilities of its wearer, a 50 to 60-year-old woman, after her big toe had been amputated, possibly because of gangrene. A glass eye with a white eyeball and a black pupil, but lacking an iris, was probably inserted into the empty eye socket of a mummy; I do not think, after everything that I have read that it would have been used by a living person.

Physicians performed other cosmetic tasks as well. Apart from prescribing various lotions and salves and unguents (which I believe are all liniments and the average person barely knows there is any difference between them) for skin care, they also produced remedies against the loss and greying of hair, which was combatted by an ointment made with blood from the horn of a black bull. Hair loss was hoped to be stopped by a mixture of honey and fats from crocodiles, lions, hippos, cats, snakes, and ibexes.

The practice of circumcision was another part of the Ancient Egyptian medicine. Unfortunately, it is difficult to estimate how pervasive that practice was. You see, the remains of mummies are of little help and literary evidence is scarce. During the New Kingdom era, both Merneptah and Ramses III had their slaughtered enemies emasculated and their genitals collected. The lack of circumcision among the Libyans and their allies is repeatedly mentioned.

The fact that they collected uncircumcised genitals as trophies may indicate that this was unusual in their eyes.

Boys destined for priesthood were circumcised as part of the initial ritual cleansing, which also included shaving their whole body. The practice of circumcision became more universal during the Late Period, perhaps as part of a rite of passage. On the other hand, female 'circumcision' (that is, clitoridectomy), an indescribable barbarity to this day, even commoner in countries of equatorial East Africa than it is in Egypt, may have been practiced occasionally, though it is thought that the only textual reference is the result of an unclear or maybe even bad translation.

The knives used in circumcision had stone blades. Flintstones and obsidian stones have edges that are sharper than modern surgical steel. It is no wonder that physicians would hesitate to replace sharp flint blades with comparatively dull metal ones, made first of bronze and later of iron. When metal instruments were finally used to any extent, they cauterized them. In some procedures, the blade was seared until it glowed red – I know you have watched at least one dramatic adventure film where a tormenting-with-a-blade scene takes place – and then used to make incisions. It cut as well as sealed up the blood vessels, limiting the bleeding.

Some Ancient Egyptians lived a very long life – to a ripe old age, as the idiom says – like Ramses II and Nitocris, the Divine Adoratrice of Amun, who reigned for more than sixty years. However, in general, the age of death surpassed the limit of 35 years only rarely. Egypt was a country that suffered from frequent floods; it was flooded for months every year. As a consequence, it was really hard not to contract bilharziasis (aka schistosomiasis). This disease is a common cause of anemia, female infertility, a weakening loss of resistance to other diseases and even death. The Ebers Papyrus addresses some of the symptoms of the disease and also some treatments and practices for prevention of bleeding in the urinal tract, which is called hematuria. Antimony disulfide is cited as the remedy of this condition in the Hearst Papyrus.

"WELLNESS": A NEW WORD FOR ANCIENT IDEAS

The Significance of Well-Reserved Papyri

The Ancient Egyptians were one of the peoples that provided modern historians with a great deal of knowledge and evidence about their attitude towards medicine and the medical knowledge that they had. This evidence has come from the numerous papyri found in archaeological searches; a great deal of our knowledge comes from the Edwin Smith Papyrus, the Ebers Papyrus and the Kahun Papyrus. They date from the 17th and 16th centuries BC, but their content is believed to be derived from even earlier sources. Archeologists found that Egyptians had fairly good knowledge about bone structure, and were aware of some of the functions of the brain and liver. This happens because unlike most prehistoric peoples, Ancient Egyptians were able to document their research and knowledge, they could read and write; and they also had a system of mathematics which helped scientists make calculations. Among other things, documented ancient Egyptian medical literature is among the oldest in existence today.

Ancient Egyptians had an agricultural economy, organized and structured government, social conventions and properly enforced laws. Their society was stable; many people lived their whole lives in the same place, unlike most of their prehistoric predecessors. This stability allowed medical research to develop. In this society, individuals were relatively wealthy, compared to their ancestors, and could afford healthcare. In Ancient Egypt, a significant number of priests became physicians. Equally, they had temples, priests, and rituals in which deceased people were mummified. In order to mummify, one had to learn something about how the human body works. In one particular mummification process, a long-hooked implement was inserted through the nostril, breaking the thin bone of the braincase, allowing the brain to be removed.

Diet and Dental Health

A restricted diet could cause or aggravate a number of ailments, some with fatal outcome. There were times when malnutrition was widespread. As their diet included much abrasive material (sand and small stone particles from grinding the corn), the teeth of elderly ancient Egyptians were often in a very poor state. To their defense, in today's industrial era, we do not know exactly what is contained in the food products we buy either.

Prehistoric dental records suggest that dental health was poor, and improved bit by bit with the increasing development of agriculture; but even in historic times when the supply of food was generally assured, the growth of the population was often stunted. Grown males reached a height of about 1.60 m and females 10 cm less during the early Middle Kingdom. Bad nutrition caused many other diseases, as well. Because of vitamin and other deficiencies, dental abrasion, and bad mouth hygiene, caries and abscesses appeared very frequently. Caries and the destruction of the enamel caused the loss of teeth at an early age and often led to death as well. Mutnodjmed, pharaoh Horemheb's second wife and sister of Nefertiti, had lost all her teeth when she died in her forties. Djedmaatesankh, a Theban musician who lived around 850 BC, suffered from 13 abscesses, extensive dental disease and a huge infected cyst, which probably killed her at the age of about 35.

Caries appeared rarely during the pre-dynastic period. It became prevalent among upper-class Egyptians as early as the Old Kingdom era. By the end of the pharaonic Egypt, it was a disease which affected all social classes. It was referred to as "a worm gnawing a tooth" which at least is comprehensible to us, and it has been suggested that they were sometimes treated by fillings made of resin and chrysocolla, a green mineral containing copper. There were also remedies for strengthening the teeth and for easing the ache in the mouth. For most of Ancient Egyptian history, there was little or no effective dental treatment available. Swollen gums were treated with a concoction of cumin, incense and onion. Opium, the toxicity of which was well known, might be given against severe pain. At times, holes were drilled into the jawbone in order to drain an abscess. As for the extraction of teeth, which might have saved the lives of many a patient, it was only rarely – if ever – practiced.

"WELLNESS": A NEW WORD FOR ANCIENT IDEAS

On the other hand, if there was no abrasive material in the food due to the circumstances, the average person would actually have a minimum incidence of caries and thus a perfect set of teeth, thanks to the paucity of sugar in the Ancient Egyptian diet. The wealthy, whose food was more refined, seem to have suffered more from caries than the poor. During Roman times, the incidence of caries appears to have grown among the population at large, possibly due to an increased consumption of sweeteners, but the level of tooth wear decreased, perhaps thanks to better sieving. The Ebers Papyrus lists a number of remedies (mostly made from herbs, such as cumin — we will study medicinal herbs in Ancient Egypt right after dentistry) dealing with teeth, although at times it is a bit unclear which is the complaint. A few examples of restorative dentistry are mentioned. One mummy was found to have three substitute teeth skillfully tied to the abutment teeth with fine gold wire, but it has been suggested that this was done post-mortem, as with prosthetics.

Since we are on it, I would like to add that the profession of the dental physician seems to have existed since early on in the third millennium. Hesy-Ra (or Hesi-re) is the first known dentist (or *Doctor of the Tooth*). But apart from this and a few other, less famous Old Kingdom instances, dentistry as a medical specialty is rarely if at all mentioned until the Greco-Roman Period.

The Pharaohs had to use dozens of drugs for each disease in order to test them and verify their effectiveness. During the Modern Kingdom, medical prescriptions were so varied that dozens of them were available for certain diseases. Therefore, a physician had to choose the most effective medication, based on prescribed criteria. Some drugs had rapid action, while others had slow action. Also, some drugs were exclusively applicable during specific seasons. For example, there was an eye medication that was exclusively used during the first two months of winter, another during the third and fourth months, and a third one was applicable all year long.

Herbal Wellness

Herbal wellness constituted a major part of ancient Egyptian medicine. The medicinal plants mentioned in the Ebers Papyrus, for instance, include opium, cannabis, myrrh, fennel, frankincense, cassia, senna, thyme, henna, juniper, aloe, linseed and castor oil – though some of the translations are a little less than certain. Cloves of garlic have been found in Egyptian burial sites, including the tomb of Tutankhamen and in the underground Serapeum of the sacred Apis bulls at Saqqara. Many herbs were steeped in wine, which was then drunk as an oral medicine.

Egyptians thought garlic and onions aided endurance, and consumed large quantities of them. Raw garlic was routinely given to asthmatics and to those suffering with bronchial-pulmonary complaints while onions helped against problems of the digestive system. Garlic was an important healing agent then just as it still is today in the Mediterranean area. Fresh cloves are peeled, mashed and macerated in a mixture of vinegar and water. This can be used to gargle and rinse the mouth, or be taken internally to treat sore throats and toothache. Another way to take garlic both for prevention as well as treatment is to macerate several cloves of mashed garlic in olive oil. Either applied as an external ointment or taken internally, it is beneficial for bronchial and lung complaints, including cold. A freshly-peeled clove of raw garlic wrapped in muslin or cheesecloth and pinned to the undergarment can protect against infectious diseases, such as colds and influenza.

Coriander was considered to have cooling, stimulant, carminative and digestive properties. Both the seeds and the plant were used as a spice in cooking to prevent and eliminate flatulence, and they were also taken as a tea for stomach and all kinds of urinary complaints, including cystitis. Coriander leaves were commonly added fresh to spicy foods to moderate their irritating effect. It was one of the herbs offered to the gods by the king, and seeds were found in the tomb of Tutankhamen and in other ancient burial sites. Cumin is an umbelliferous herb indigenous to Egypt. Its seeds were considered to be stimulants and effective against flatulence. They were often used together with coriander for flavoring. Cumin powder mixed with some wheat flour as a binder and a little water was applied to relieve the pain of any arthritic or aching joints. Powdered cumin mixed with grease or lard was inserted as an anal suppository to disperse heat from the anus and stop itching. Leaves from many plants, such as willow, sycamore, and acacia, were used in poultices. Tannic acid derived from acacia seeds commonly helped for lowering the temperature of the vessels and heal burns. Castor oil, figs, and dates were used as laxatives. In case you are wondering, all the information in the last few paragraphs on herbs has come from the already-several-times mentioned Ebers Papyrus.

Exceptional Facts

Ancient Egyptian physicians knew that the body had a pulse, and that it was associated with the function of the heart. They had a very basic knowledge of the cardiac system, but overlooked the phenomenon of blood circulating around the body — either because they missed it, or thought it did not matter, they were unable to distinguish blood vessels, nerves, or tendons. The ancient Egyptians were traders, and travelled long distances, coming back with herbs and spices from faraway lands. Their relatively high standard of living gave them free time, which they could use for observing things and thinking about them; and it is widely known that medical research involves much patience and observation.

Trepanation, practiced in many early cultures for a number of reasons, is not mentioned in any of the medical papyri, but seems to have been performed occasionally with the use of a mallet and a chisel. Fourteen skulls, some wholly healed and some partially healed, have been found. Limb amputations were also performed.

Tapeworms, or *the snakes in the belly*, as they are mentioned in the Hearst Papyrus, were dealt with by an infusion of pomegranate root in water, which was strained and drunk. The alkaloids contained in it paralyzed the worms' nervous system, and the latter pulled away. Ulcers were treated with yeast, as were stomach ailments. Some of the medicines were made from plant materials imported from abroad. Mandrake introduced from Canaan was thought to be an aphrodisiac and, mixed with alcohol, induced unconsciousness. Cedar oil, an antiseptic, originated in the Levant. The Persian henna was grown in Egypt since the Middle Kingdom, and – if identical with *henu* mentioned in the Ebers Papyrus – was used against hair loss. Catarrh was treated with aloe, which came from Eastern Africa. Frankincense, containing tetrahydrocannabinol and used like hashish as a painkiller, was imported from Punt.

Ancient Egyptians used various minerals and animal products, as well. Honey and grease were part of many wound treatments, mother's milk was occasionally given against viral diseases like the common cold, fresh meat laid on open wounds and sprains, and animal dung was thought to be effective at times. A cosmetics jar at the Cairo Museum bears the caption: "Eye lotion to be dispersed, good for eyesight." An Egyptian papyrus from 1500 BCE includes recipes for treating conjunctivitis and cornea, iris, and eyelid problems. Lead-based chemicals like carbonates and acetates were popular for their therapeutic properties. Malachite was used as an eyeliner and had therapeutic value. In a country where eye infections were endemic, the effects of its germicidal qualities were appreciated even if the reasons for its effectiveness were not understood.

Saqqara is an ancient burial ground in Egypt, serving as the necropolis for the Ancient Egyptian capital, Memphis. In it, there is the tomb of Ankhmahor, known as The Physician's Tomb. In one of its wall pictures, two men are having their extremities treated in various ways explained as manicure, massage or surgery. In the accompanying text, the patient implores the physician to not cause him any pain. At any rate, people at least occasionally survived surgery. Bodies of amputees from as early as the Old and Middle Kingdoms have been found which display signs of healing. Prostheses which show signs of wear and tear, have also been discovered. The reasons for these amputations are unknown and none of the surviving medical texts mention the possibility of, let alone reasons for amputation as a therapeutic treatment. Lastly, poppies are occasionally mentioned in Ancient Egyptian medical literature, so the physicians of the era must have had a pretty good idea of their properties.

Furthermore, Ancient Egyptian physicians were sought after by kings and queens from faraway lands because they were considered to be the best in the world. Now, as far as their practices are concerned, there are a few comments to be made. On the one hand, some of their recommendations were fairly proper – they advised people to wash and shave their bodies as measures to prevent infections. They also advised people to eat carefully, and to avoid unclean animals and raw fish. On the other hand, some of their practices were strange and most likely did more harm than good. Several medical prescriptions contained animal dung, which might have useful molds and fermentation substances, but were also infested with bacteria and must have caused many serious infections.

The Classification of Physicians

Let's now put a few pieces of information about Ancient Egyptian physicians into time perspective, shall we? The ancient Egyptian texts of the Old Kingdom of Egypt (2635-2155 BC) mention at least 50 physicians, the sources being mainly tombs. Though most physicians were men, female physicians existed as well and they had distinct titles. The earliest record of a physician was Hesy-Ra (2700 BC), who was "Chief of Dentists and Doctors" to King Dioser, while the first female physician was probably Peseshet (2400 BC), who was known as the supervisor of all female physicians. The hierarchy was pretty clear and specific. The top doctors worked in the royal court and, below them, there were inspectors who would supervise the proper actions of all medical practitioners. There were also specialized doctors, such as proctologists, gastroenterologists, dentists, and ophthalmologists. In particular, a proctologist was called *nery phuyt* which meant "shepherd of the anus".

Physicians were literate, some were scribes and others were priests at the same time. Most inherited the profession from their fathers but needed to be trained in the field. As I said, the profession was organized hierarchically right from the start and it remained that way later on, as well; just the titles had naturally changed. More precisely, the Chief Physician was at the top and was followed by titles, such as Master of Physicians, Director of Physicians, Inspector of Physicians, Plain Physician and auxiliaries such as Bandage personnel etc. Texts deal with diagnosis, treatments and prescriptions. Plus, surgery and mummification processes used by Ancient Egyptians still amaze modern experts.

All major and expected diseases were known and treated, ailments were attributed to spirits, ghosts and revenge by gods and goddesses. Texts dealing with gynecology cover fertility, sterility, pregnancy, contraception and abortion. Women were tested to decide whether they could conceive or not. Their treatments were based on examination, followed by diagnosis. Descriptions of the examination — which, by the way, is the most fundamental part of the job — are lengthier than both the diagnosis or the recommended treatment in most papyri. The pots containing medicines were (at least occasionally) labeled, stating the remedy's composition and how to use it. One label in particular that has been found indicates that the pot contains saw dust, acacia leaves, galena, and goose fat and that it must be used as bandage. Acacia tree products and galena were frequently used to treat eye complaints.

Concerning their treatment plans, Ancient Egyptian physicians were conservative: If no remedy was known for a particular condition, then they only chose steps that would probably not endanger the patient in any way. Some head wounds, for instance, that were considered as conditions better not to be treated, an ointment would be anointed externally forestalling possible further infections. Egyptian theories and practices influenced the Greeks, who furnished many of the physicians in the Roman Empire, and through them, they also influenced the Arab and European medical thought for centuries to come.

However, the Egyptians were behind Babylonian doctors who had gone further and designed the first pregnancy test known in history. That test involved placing in the women's vagina a tampon impregnated with the juice of various plants in an alum solution. This was left in position either overnight or for three days. Pregnancy or non-pregnancy was

"WELLNESS": A NEW WORD FOR ANCIENT IDEAS

indicated by colour changes between red and green. The test used the pH value of the woman's vaginal secretions. However, the truth is that rational thinking and sound medical observation were used not alone but alongside magic and sorcery.

The part of Ancient Egyptian medical history that I find regrettable is that much of the pharmacopoeia and many medical practices were ineffective, if not downright deleterious. For instance, excrement used in medicines will only extremely rarely prove to be a wholesome choice, and if applied as wound dressing, it will probably cause tetanus poisoning, yet dung continued to be used in Europe until the Middle Ages. The reliance on magic and faith might be the main reason for the delay in developing more rational views of the causes of diseases and their cures. On the other hand, the strong belief of the patient in the divine origins of the cure probably played a large part in its being effective and, in the absence of something better, more secure and more reliant, often the only support a physician could give were the natural healing processes.

According to Ancient Egyptian physicians, — perhaps I should start referring to them as AEP by now for short — there were three (main) types of injuries. Obviously, there were the treatable and the untreatable ones. The treatable ones were dealt with immediately, while for the untreatable ones the physician did not even make an effort; once the ailment was deemed untreatable, they would not intervene. As for the third type of injury, it concerns the contestable ones, that is the not life-threatening ones. In this case, the patient would be put under medical observation and the physicians would decide in their own time when and how they should intervene. Well, if the patient was still alive, of course. A condition that is not life-threatening for most people might be for someone. If this is true today, it was even truer back then.

Magic VS. Logic

Earlier we talked about magic and divine punishment, as everyday life in Egypt involved beliefs and fear of magic, gods, evil spirits and the such. Magic was based on the assumption that an object with certain qualities, or an action of a certain kind, could be used to create an action of positive energy (healing) or to repel something evil. Magical elements are mentioned in medical texts; they were added to the prescriptions and the treatments for diseases. The religious and magic rituals probably had a powerful placebo effect, which was perceived as proof of the rituals' effectiveness. Anthropologists, archeologists, and medical historians say there did not appear to be a clear difference between a priest and a doctor in those days. For some conditions, like sterility and impotence in men, magic was widely used while other, easier conditions relied mainly on some medicinal treatment.

As it naturally went in every civilization, religion gave place to logic. The religious procedures were gradually replaced by more and more tangible treatments. Some healing treatments used medicinal products or plants or herbs that looked similar to the illness they were treating. For instance, ostrich eggs were used to treat a fractured skull. This practice is known as *simila similibus* (which means "similar with similar"). It is a practice that existed on a global scale and still exists in modern alternative medicine. Today, this is what we call homeopathy, as you may have guessed.

The heart was extensively studied. It is unclear, however, whether the blood circulation in the arteries was fully understood. In fact, the heart was considered to be the organ of reason instead of the brain, though the latter was studied extensively as well. Ancient papyri inform us that Ancient Egyptians were discovering little by little things about how the human body works and that they knew how important pulse rates, blood and air were to the workings of the human body. A physician could say with certainty that a patient had some problem just by auscultating them to find a weak heartbeat. In general, anatomy was well-understood, with dissection being a common procedure.

Among all those precious well-preserved papyri that have helped us paint a clear picture of what was going on in Ancient Egypt not just socially but from every aspect, the Papyrus Ebers is probably the most significant one. At least medicine-wise, it is a real treasure; It is a document that actually gives names to vital organs such as the spleen, the heart, the anus, the lungs et cetera.

Another papyrus, the Edwin Smith Papyrus, includes a description of the brain in much detail. This document shows that the brain was very well researched considering the few means they had at the time. It is probable that they reached to this level of knowledge concerning the brain because of the practice they had of embalming dead bodies. The work of an embalmer was thoroughly described by Herodotus who was Greek of course, but visited Egypt in the 5th century BC. Apparently, they cut along the side of the body, took out the abdomen and filled the cavity with spices, such as myrrh and cassia. Then, they put the body in natron for 70 days. Those organs that were removed in the embalming process, were put in some kind of jar along with preserving spices, and put into the tomb of the deceased. Though religious law forbade the embalmers from studying the bodies of the dead, it is almost certain they would have gained some knowledge of the human anatomy simply from the work that they did.

Hygiene

During my research, I was thrilled to discover how important personal cleanliness and appearance were in Egyptian everyday life. You know, us women, we love our hygiene. The provision of water so that people can wash themselves, their animals, and their houses was a vital part of preventing diseases from spreading. The general aim of Ancient Egyptian public health was to protect the community from diseases and to keep everybody as healthy as possible. However, I was not so thrilled when I found out that cleanliness was promoted for social and religious reasons, and not health ones. But since they are not with us anymore, I am going to let this one slide.

Their houses were only equipped with rudimentary baths and toilets. There was no public health infrastructure as we know it, with sewage systems, proper medical care and public hygiene. Most people used mosquito nets during the hot months, although it is not certain as of yet whether they did that to protect themselves against malaria and other diseases, or simply because they did not want to be bitten. Many people even wore make-up around their eyes as a way of protection from various diseases. As for priests, they washed themselves, their clothing, and their eating utensils on a regular basis. But I have to tell you that they did it for religious reasons. Although hygiene practices did help protect their health, this was not the real reason; cleanliness was an appeal to their gods.

Taking the Zoroastrian teachings into consideration, it is not surprising that the famous, historically documented Achaemenid Medical School was founded and financed by Darius the Great (522-486 BC) in Egypt. It was located next to the temple of Neith and was named Saiis. Once the students had graduated, they would spread all over the empire and practice medicine. The Egyptian director of the school, Ujahorus, was himself a scientist. On his statue that is maintained in the Vatican, the following words have been inscribed: "Darius the Great King ordered that I shall return to Egypt and rebuild the Neith Temple... I provided books and educated the youth and brought them instruments. He realized the value of medical science and for every patient that I saved, he reveres and prays to God." It is interesting that on a papyrus discovered in Egypt, the following words are written: "I have come out of the Saiis", indicating the pride a physician took in the university from which he graduated.

CURING WARRIOR WOUNDS IN GREECE

Hippocrates: «Ουκ ένι ιατρικήν είδέναι, όστις μη οίδεν ό τι εστίν άνθρωπος.»
"It is impossible for anyone to know medicine who does not know what man is."

"...But save me. Take me to the ship, cut this arrow out of my leg, wash the blood from it with warm water and put the right things on it - the plants they say you have learned about from Achilles who learned them from Chiron, the best of the Centaurs."
—The Iliad of Homer, Book XI

▍ Disease Meant Divine Punishment: A Karmic View!

Health in Ancient Greece was considered a supreme good of paramount value and so every different human age was dedicated to a protector-god. The title is just a sort of clickbait; medicine was as widely extended as one would expect. There were many established hygiene measures concerning the drying out of swamps and also the water supply and the sewerage system of urban settlements. It appears that there were public doctors in many cities for the protection of public health and that the state provided medical care to the needy for free, having imposed a special medical poll tax, the *"iatrikon."* This practice was not in force in Athens, where Plato deterred his people from taking drugs, recommending physiotherapy instead.

Disease in Ancient Greece was seen as the body's natural reaction to the mistakes of the soul. It was regarded as a reaction of the defense system with the aim to get the soul back on the right track, to make it follow God's path again. God's path is the contact with nature, the understanding of nature's causalities, the most important one being the balance between opposites. When a person is sick, the human soul falls off God's divine path which is the beginning of everything, the "one" in a binary reality where humans must live and find the right equilibrium. Disease was widely assumed to be the result of divine displeasure, transgressions of various kinds, or magical forces. Diagnosis might involve prayer, interpreting animal entrails, or determining how the patient had transgressed. This mix of magico-religious medicine was also part of the Greek reality during the Hippocratic period.

So, the human soul had to face the evil, but without eradicating it because the evil is part of the human nature. On the other hand, the sick individual must not let the evil dominate either, because in this case the evil will destroy the soul, obviously. The human soul has to find the right balance between food and movement. Food is the earthly element, the bad, the joy, the pleasure, the ego, and everything that is related to those. Movement is the celestial, the good, the fatigue, the effort, the pain, the sorrow, the "we," and everything that is related to those. When the soul has managed to find the right balance in that binary world, then the body is of excellent health and the individual is alive and well. When this balance is lost, the body gets sick and everything that is bad prevails.

I always try to present both sides of a story, both the (seemingly) positive and the (seemingly) negative. Therefore, I have to say that the distinction between the spiritual and physical worlds is often a blurred line in Ancient Greek medicine. There is an oxymoron even as far as the Ancient Greek God of Medicine is concerned; Asclepius was considered to be a dispenser of healing and, at the same time, a highly-skilled medical practitioner. He was called upon by patients at his many sanctuaries to give them medical advice in their dreams and then, the patients' physicians could act upon the given information. Grateful patients even went as far as to leave monuments at the site, which revealed some of the problems that needed to be treated, including blindness, limping, snakebites, infection, and aphasia, among other disorders.

The History of Ancient Greek Medicine: A Brief Presentation

The very start of Greek Medicine can be found in the myths of Ancient Greeks concerning the genealogical trees of Greek Gods. Apollo is the one who can be considered as the founder of medicine, or at least of medical thought. His moniker Paeonian is derived from the verb «παίω» which means "to cure." Other Paeonian Gods, and therefore curators, were Artemis (twin sister of Apollo), Athena, and Asclepius. The presence of a midwife at the birth of the God of Medicine shows that both medicine and treatment come from midwifery and maternity care.

It is interesting and noteworthy that Apollo was the Greek God of the Sun and the Light, among other things, and that he represented sunlight on Earth. This means that Ancient Greeks recognized the light of the sun as a primordial curative force. And thanks to Greece's particular geomorphology, the sunlight diffused in this country is notably beneficial to humans, something that can serve as an explanation for all the intellectual and material accomplishments of Ancient Greeks (and for modern-day tourism blooming). However, Greeks had understood that medical art is a human intellectual accomplishment and believed that, as such, it could disrespect the natural causalities, which brightly reveals the big size of human arrogance.

As Plutarch put it amazingly in words in his body of work *Moralia*, "For as regards the care of the body, men have discovered two sciences, the medical and the gymnastic, of which the one implants health, the other sturdiness, in the body; but for the illnesses and affections of the mind, philosophy alone is the remedy." More generally, one could argue that Ancient Greek medicine was a compilation of many theories and practices, a collection that is a little bit diverse, constantly expanding through new ideologies, new trials, new experiments, new knowledge. Those could be acquired with practice or come from other countries, such as Egypt and the Roman Empire. Many elements in AG medicine intertwined the spiritual with the physical.

Specifically, the theories and ideologies from which ancient Greek medicine derived included the humors, gender, geographic location, social class, diet, trauma (injury, wound), beliefs, and mindset of the patient. From early on, Ancient Greeks believed that illnesses were nothing but divine punishments and that healing was, quite literally, a gift from the gods. It was theorized that gender played a role in medicine because some diseases and treatments were different for women than for men. Moreover, the geographic location, the season of the year, and the social class affected the living conditions of people and put them through different environmental issues, such as mosquitoes, rats, and availability of clean potable water. Nevertheless, common threads running through Greek medical thought included a preoccupation about the positive and negative effects of an individual's diet and the belief that the patient could actually do something to help their health status, in contrast with the more fatalistic and spiritual mindset of earlier times. There was significant focus on the beliefs and mentality of the patient in the diagnosis and treatment theories.

In addition, it was recognized that the mind played a role in healing, or that it might also be the sole basis for the illness, in some cases. So, the notion of mental wellbeing was perceived early on. Diet was considered an issue as well in cases there was no access to adequate, proper nourishment. Traumas, such as that suffered by warriors, caused from dog bites or other injuries, played a role in theories relating to understanding anatomy and infections.

If anyone knows anything about Ancient Greek history, it is that wars were a pretty common phenomenon. In the Homeric Epics, references are made to various techniques used to relieve the pain of soldiers injured or amputated in war. In Hippocratic medicine, pain is considered to be caused by disorders in the balance of the four humors or by external factors, such as weather conditions, distress, nutrition, and accidents. Special pharmacological substances were used to manage it, as well as the method of opposites.

We are lucky that the use of many substances, derived mostly from plants, has been well-recorded. These natural medicinal substances can cause analgesia, narcosis, dizziness, or partial unconsciousness, when administered alone or as part of a wrong combination. For the treatment of war wounds and amputations, medical preparations and ingredients were taken right from the nature and they included seawater, rainwater, and honey. Medicinal herbs and plants in the form of powder and vinegar were also used.

There are also records that indicate treatment practices on war wounds during the Trojan War and even treatment of infected wounds. Treating wounded soldiers was actually one of the best ways for a doctor to learn his trade and widen his knowledge of the human body and its internal functions. What's more, in contrast to other patients, treating a soldier was probably less risky for the practitioner in case things went wrong, because his wounds were caused in war and not by a possibly contagious disease. Aside from the health problems that may have affected civilians, such as malnutrition, dehydration, hypothermia, fever and typhoid, the soldiers-treating doctors had to deal with wounds made by swords, spears, javelins, arrows and projectiles from slings.

Surgery and Surgical Instruments

Medical practitioners knew very well the importance of removing foreign bodies, such as arrow heads, from the wound and the necessity to properly clean the wound right after that. Which is why they started making the arrowheads barbed; they wanted them to be more difficult to remove and therefore more lethal. Greek doctors knew that it was important to stop excessive blood loss as soon as possible in order to prevent hemorrhage (although they also thought that blood-flowing could be beneficial too). Concerning surgery, it may also have included the use of opium as an anesthetic, although the many references in literature to patients being held down during surgery suggest otherwise; that the use of anesthetic was rare, that is.

Following the operation, they closed the wounds with the use of stitches of flax or linen thread and the wound dressed with linen bandages or sponges, sometimes soaked in water, wine, oil or vinegar. Leaves could also be used for the same purpose and wounds would also be sealed using egg-white or honey. Post-operation treatment was also considered important – the importance of diet, for example, or the use of plants with anti-inflammatory properties, such as celery.

Hippocrates noticed the separation of limb gangrene and made incisions between dead and alive tissue to treat the condition. Hippocrates's views were highly innovative for his time, as he suggested chest tube output for possible liquid in external fixation and traction when aligning broken bones. He believed that the wounds must be kept dry in order to be properly and quickly healed. In addition, the formation of pus was considered a positive factor for the reduction of wound complications because of the frequent occurrence of infections. As a consequence, the combined findings of Hippocrates and Galen had an influence on surgical care practices of injuries and wounds until the Middle Ages.

Over time, Greek physicians managed to acquire a basic knowledge of the human anatomy, assisted undoubtedly by the observation of grievously wounded soldiers and, from the 4th century BC, through animal dissection as well. However, some claimed that this was useless, because they believed that the inner body got altered once it came in contact with air and light. Others – just like in our days – protested that using animals for such purposes was pure cruelty. Human dissection would have to wait until the Hellenistic times when such discoveries as the full nervous system were made. Nevertheless, there was an increasing urge to discover what made a healthy body function well rather than what had made an unhealthy one break down. The lack of practical knowledge, though, did result in some fundamental mistakes, such as the idea proposed in the treatise *On Ancient Medicine* (5th century BC) that physical pain arises from the body's inability to assimilate certain foods.

"WELLNESS": A NEW WORD FOR ANCIENT IDEAS

By 500 BC, Greek physicians became more interested in using scientific observation and logic to figure out what were the causes of diseases and what they could do to fight them. It took some time, but they managed to work out a logical system for a better understanding of disease. The main collection of writings on Greek medicine is, of course, Hippocrates's body of work. This logical system began with the idea of humors, which was popular all over Europe and Asia at the time (in India and China, as well as Greece). The idea of humors may even have gotten started in Greece, where it makes its earliest appearance.

Well, the – subjective – way I see it, Greek medical practice may have included errors, perhaps many of them, and perhaps even a few fatal ones, but we should admit that Greek practitioners had started practicing the medical profession in the right direction. Observation, experience and experimentation meant that those who followed in Hellenistic and Roman times, such as Galen and Aulus Cornelius Celsus (or simply Celsus), could continue their enquiries along the long and winding road towards greater and more accurate scientific knowledge of the human body, the diseases and ailments it is susceptible to, and the potential that the available cures can provide.

Of course, to operate, a surgeon needs not only the necessary knowledge but also the appropriate medical instruments. And in Ancient Greece, there was an impressive abundance of useful instruments for surgery and medical practice. Most of them were discovered and came into light during the excavation of the Surgeon's Tomb in the eastern necropolis of New Paphos in the island of Cyprus. This large necropolis called *The Tombs of the Kings* lies about two kilometers west of Paphos. Some of those instruments were: scalpels, stone palettes, fleams, dirks with handles, cauterizing knives, various types of scissors, forceps, sharp hooks, stirrups, fine needles, bivalvular speculums, hysteroscopes, catheters, enemas, drainage cannulas, measuring spoons, as well as various toolkits for the above.

The 4 Elements & The 4 Humors: How interconnected are they?

The main wellness theory that influenced medicine in Ancient Greece was that of fire («πυρ») and water («ύδωρ»). I really hope that you can perceive the similarity between the Modern English words and their Greek etymological mothers. In Ancient Greek medical thought, there is the idea that everything in nature begins from two opposite yet complementary forces, which coexist in all phenomena as the primary cores of movement and structure, and that idea is pretty consistent. I'd like to make it easy for you and tell you right away that the fire & water theory in Ancient Greece corresponds fairly well with the yin & yang theory in Eastern Asia, that we already studied in the first chapter.

Another theory, or to put it more correctly, the evolved version of the aforementioned theory of fire and water is the theory of the Four Elements. Those are again fire and water, plus air and earth. This theory came to be even more influential than its predecessor and became the basis of Ancient Greeks' thought of medicine. So, it is only appropriate to present this essential theory right away, before going any further. The four humors/elements theories provided a theoretical framework that lasted through the centuries.

The first ones to speak of nature's elements in general are the Ionian philosophers in the 6th century BC: Thales, Anaximenes, Anaximander, Heraclitus, and of course Pythagoras. The latter was the one to formulate the Four Elements theory, after having been taught by his predecessors. Hippocrates was also influenced by the Pythagorean thought concerning the four elements. In essence, the entire Hippocratic theory of the 4 humors is based upon that of the 4 elements. The humors are the 4 elements of nature inside the human body. After all, Hippocrates comes from Cos, an Aegean island next to the Ionia coastline, where the Ionian thought flourishes in the 6th century BC. Plato and Aristotle are also on the same wavelength. As Hippocrates puts it, the only way to be initiated in the theory of the Four Elements is through observation of the natural events. Besides, my Greek antecedents were

"WELLNESS": A NEW WORD FOR ANCIENT IDEAS

physiocrats (naturalists). Nature was everyone's primordial teacher and only the things that could be verified in the natural reality were true in their core; this was the norm of the Ancient Greek way of thinking. Observing nature is the only necessary and complete way to go.

Let's now meet our four elements, beginning with fire. The main representative of fire is the Sun. Other representatives of the universal fire are the stars we see in a star-studded sky; although in essence, stars are suns too and their distance from the Earth makes us see them as little glinting sparks. So, what one has to observe in order to familiarize themselves with the element of Fire is the Sun, its equinoxes, its solstices, and its daily cycle. Observing the Moon also helps us understand the element of Fire and at the same time, that of Water. the Moon emits a light that is the reflection of the sunlight (which is emitted in all directions). The moonlight is colder, since it can lighten up a place but cannot warm us like the sunlight does. In reality, the "cold" moonlight seems to affect the movement of the planet's waters and cause tides (periodic rises and falls of large bodies of water). Observing the Moon means observing it in the celestial sphere and knowing the lunar phases, such as the new moon, the full moon, the first quarter, the last quarter, the waning crescent, et cetera. Lastly, there are also other suns in the universe, whose distance is incredibly immense, still they do have an impact on the Earth. The latter too has sources of fire. Apart from the sources of fire coming from the sky, there is also a source of fire coming from the earth and that is the lava erupting from volcanoes. Observing all of the above leads us to the conclusion that fire can take many forms, but it is basically one united element.

If we want to understand the nature of the element of Air, we have to observe its movements. In fact, the air expresses the very concept of moving, despite the fact that the air movement's generating force is fire. The air becomes the host of the fire's movement and can blow in all possible directions. What we have to observe is the air's direction and hue. There are no unwinnable obstacles for the air. The air can overcome it all; it is simply a matter of time. Actually, the obstacles make it even stronger and more sweeping. This phenomenon is also observed in the vessels and the veins of the human body. When the humors flow and come across an obstacle, such as an atherosclerotic plaque, the "blast" of air produced by that flow is reinforced. This can lead to either an increased blood pressure or an arterial murmur. The air has three significant characteristics: fluidity, variability, and a tendency to take up all of the available space. The air leaves no empty space; it fills up everything, everywhere. Variability itself entails adjustability. The air's tendency to occupy all of the space is a quality that is transferred as it is when the four elements are created, that is when life itself is created. This is the reason why the element of Air is identified with that of wood in the Chinese Five Elements theory. This quality of the air is expressed as an expansionary, imperialistic behavior when it comes to human beings. So, anything that has to do with expansiveness on a mental or physical level shows the presence, and perhaps the excessiveness, of air.

Thirdly, let's pay a visit to the element of Water. If we want to understand water's nature, we have to observe that the water's condition differs depending on the intensity of the element of Fire. Therefore, in extremely high temperatures (fire excess), water turns into air (evaporation), while in extremely low temperatures (freezing/coagulation), water turns into earth (ice). It is also important that water can activate seeds, hence the human egg is activated and expressed in watery conditions (vaginal humidity) and develops within them (amniotic fluids etc.). Water tends to move downwards; it is an earthly material that obeys the rule of gravity. It also has the tendency to be united with itself; it has an introverted behavior. We attest this behavior on more than 70% of the planet, that is the latter's bodies of water (oceans, seas, lakes, rivers, streams, etc.). The human body consists of the same proportion of earth and water. We often say that the earth feeds us but it is true that water's presence is indispensable in order for the introverted process of alimentation to push through. So, when a damaging factor, such as cold, enters the body through the process of nutrition (ice cream, for example), it will tend to enter more internal levels of the body and be trapped in them for long. Lastly, during certain natural phenomena (low-pressure systems, full moons, and south winds), water is inflated and acquires fullness. So, when someone already has increased humidity in their body during said phenomena, they may have a feeling of heaviness all over their body or in some parts of it, a feeling of swelling, or feel pain. On the contrary, when water is shrunk, consumed, that is, when there is a lack of humidity, aridity appears and consequently the elements of Fire and Air are increased. This is what Chinese medicine describes as yin deficiency and yang excess.

The element of Earth is the fourth and final one of the studied theory. The earth has mass and weight; it is a physical substance. The earthy materials of the Earth, including the water, exert a gravitational pulling force, which attracts light (Fire), warmness (Air), and all the other materials that surround it, such as comets and water. The nature of soil is such that it can only pull the other elements through gravity. And at the same time, it tries to trap them inside it. The earth's gravitational pull is transferred as a quality to all living things. Female beings express mainly the energy-related behavior of water and earth while male beings mostly express that of fire and air. The physical expression of the earth and water's behavior in female beings is basically the latter's genital organs. For instance, a woman's uterus tries in every way to attract and hold in it the male sperm just like water and earth do with fire and air through their gravitational pulling force. The earth has some further features. These are stability, dryness and coldness. The element of Earth also has a diversity and a diversification that are caused exactly because the other three elements can be in different conditions during the earth's production procedure. This diversity greatly affects the life of humans. The four elements create the various geo-climatological conditions around the world. Apart from its internal composition, they also create the earth's various forms: mountains, valleys, deserts, plateaus, creeks, canyons, et cetera. Humans are equally diverse and different. There is no stone identical to another stone, just as every human being is unique and different.

Now, let's see how the four humors are related to those four elements. Firstly, the sanguine humor (the blood) is related to the element of Air and to the liver. It dictated courage, hope and love. The choleric humor (the yellow bile) is associated with the element of

Fire and the gallbladder. If in excess, it could lead to bad temper and anger. The melancholic humor (the black bile) is related to the element of Earth and to the spleen. In case it dominated the body, it could lead to sleeplessness and irritation. Finally, the phlegmatic humor (the phlegm) is associated with the element of Water and the brain. It was responsible for rationality, but it would also dull the emotions if allowed to become the dominant element in an individual's body.

Phlegm might seem the sign of a common cold to us, but for the Hippocratics it was one of four humors which were constitutive of health and disease, and thus at the heart of the Hippocratic physiology and pathology. As for the centrality of the brain that is now a commonplace in scientific thinking, it was not so with the Greeks. Plato followed Hippocrates in viewing the brain as the seat of psychological activity, but Plato's pupil Aristotle believed that the heart is the center of emotion and other mental functions.

The Confluence Between Diet and Health: They Do Meet Somewhere!

In this part, we will examine the dietary habits of Ancient Greeks that helped in unpleasant health situations. They understood that the body's wellness depended, among other things, on one's diet as well. Ancient Greeks used to eat many fermented foods, such as pickles, yogurt, beer, kale, and cheese made from non-pasteurized milk. During the fermentation process, carbohydrates such as starch and sugar transform into acids, like lactic acid which provides many beneficial bacteria for our body. Eating foods that have undergone zymosis (i.e. fermentation) is good for our immune system, while giving us abundant vitamins, such as Vitamin B and K2. It also helps us clear our bodies from toxins, lose weight, and fight autoimmune diseases. Moreover, our intestine produces more serotonin, which is a neurotransmitter that has a positive impact on our mood and behavior.

Ancient Greeks ate many fruit and vegetables as well. Many varieties of apples, quinces, plums, grapes were consumed often, with figs and caprifigs being their favorite kind of fruit. As for vegetables,

"WELLNESS": A NEW WORD FOR ANCIENT IDEAS

legumes, and herbs, they grew garlic, onions, horse beans, green beans, peas, lettuce, lupins, bulbs, lentils, and chickpeas. Equally, they searched for mushrooms, fennel, asparagus, and other herbs in river's ends and wild fields. They grew vegetables not just to eat them but also for their healthful effect. There are references where Attalus I, the ruler of Pergamum, who grew henbane, hellebore, and conium in his vegetable garden, interested in their poisonous action, so we see that herbs were used malevolently as well.

Furthermore, numerous herbs and spices much loved by (either ancient or modern) Greeks were used in medicine, something we will study as well. Lastly, let's not forget the royal jelly that, according to the ancient religious tradition, was the food of the Olympian Gods; the substance that made them immortal. After much research, it was found to have a positive effect on various neurological, psychiatric, and cardiovascular diseases, on the fields of pediatrics, geriatrics, ophthalmology, stomatology, dermatology, hematology, and gynecology, and on disorders of the urinary system.

How Were the Medical Professions Perceived?

Ancient Greeks took the matter of disease very seriously. Disease led to the death of many people and very often at a very young age. About one out of three babies died because of some disease whose cure was not known yet — I have talked about this in the prologue, so I am not going to repeat any more of this horrible, devastating information. Therefore, they took equally seriously the medical professions and anyone who practiced them; they kind of had to, really. In the late 6th century BC, two Greek city-states were famous for their doctors, those of Croton (in Southern Italy) and Cyrene (in Northern Africa). But in the 5th century the most famous centers were Cos, the birthplace of Hippocrates, and Cnidus, just opposite Cos on the mainland of Asia Minor (aka Anatolia). They created and developed prospering medical schools. These schools became the main centers for teaching medicine, and the physicians associated with either place shared certain medical practices. The instruction in these schools was very informal, compared to today. No set term was established concerning the period of training that a medical student should undergo, nor did they obtain a certificate of their right to practice medicine at the end. As far as we know, no legal or general method existed to prevent an amateur, an inadequately trained apprentice, or a quack from practicing it. Their establishing themselves as doctors did not depend on how they had been trained, but on their own conscience, on the reputation they acquired in practice, and also by keeping the confidence of their clients. However, this was not as alarming as it may sound, since the apprentice system they applied was a self-policing one. More precisely, each of the masters (physicians) would watch carefully each one of their apprentices to make sure they were able to adequately do their job. At the same time, the structural political fragmentation of the Greek territory into hundreds of independent states made almost impossible for a practicing physician not to be checked upon concerning their profession. And of course, attendance at one of the renowned medical schools, such as that of Cos, would provide evidence as to the physician's qualifications.

So, in a nutshell, seeing that there was no official qualification evidence for medical practitioners, anyone could set themselves up as a physician and travel around looking for patients on whom to practice the art of medicine, until being caught in some way. On the other hand, in Sparta, they had a specific and specialized medical personnel that was responsible for healthcare within the Spartan professional army.

In the beginning, authorities in Ancient Greece were not aware of the need for an organized public health system. The Greek city-states did not put any effort to ensure that their people had an adequate supply of clean water to wash themselves and keep their homes clean. There was no public sewage system either. But, the Greek people felt that they had to stay clean and healthy. Especially the rich and the educated saw to it that they cleaned their teeth, washed regularly, ate healthy food and kept being fit by exercising on a daily basis. According to Hippocrates, poor people would be too focused on making ends meet and could not afford to be too concerned about their overall health on the same level. As we will see, Greeks also tried to keep their four bodily humors in balance. And, of course, living in moderation was another daily aim of utter importance.

However, though they had no official qualification, medical practitioners do seem to have generally enjoyed a high social regard, just thanks to their indispensable-for-living profession. As Homer states in the Iliad (11.514-15), "a doctor is worth many other men when it comes to cutting out arrows and spreading soothing drugs on wounds." Not only did doctors give medical advice and treatments, but other groups too could utilize their practical experience, such as midwives and gym trainers.

Hippocrates – Part I

As a Greek – and a proud one, I should add – I have two words, that is Medicine and Hippocrates, inextricably linked in my mind and conscience. And I know for sure I am not the only one. Hippocrates is referred to as the "Father of (Western) Medicine" having prescribed professional practices for physicians through his aforementioned oath. I put the word "western" in parentheses because it is very often omitted. So, a tribute to this highly distinguished science personality is only appropriate, if not absolutely imposed.

Hippocrates was a Greek physician who lived during the Golden Age of Athens, in the fifth century BC (460 – 370 BC). His contributions to the scientific field of medicine, especially as the founder of the Hippocratic School of Medicine, were tremendous, almost inexhaustible. He served as an unparalleled model for physicians and coined the Hippocratic oath, which is still relevant as it has always been and in global use. If this is not a magnificent life achievement, I do not know what is. He vastly advanced and brought forward the systematic study of clinical medicine as well, summing up the medical knowledge of previous schools. However, I should also mention that the oath did not include any requirements about respecting patient autonomy. For example, the oath did not say anything about giving patients the power to control decisions about their final care. It also didn't require physicians to tell the truth to their patients or disclose diagnostic and prognostic information.

Hippocrates of Cos was possibly the first person to argue that having a disease or being ill is a natural human thing and not something associated with superstitions or provoked by gods, demons or any other divine, mythological creatures. He was credited by the disciples of Pythagoras of making a logical and prudent connection between medicine and philosophy. At the same time, he was the one who separated medicine from religion, seeing the two as distinct parts of human nature. I want you to take a minute here and try to realize what used to go through humanity's minds millennia ago. Getting sick (as in vomiting) after having eaten a tomato meant that the... tomato-eater was punished by Zeus for some less than good action they had done, like having stolen that tomato from their neighbor's field crops, for example. The fact that there might have been a worm in that tomato was not even a possibility; not even close to be seen and accepted as a possibility. So, yes, before Hippocrates' writings, Greeks considered illness pretty much as a spiritual malady, that was caused and that would also be cured according to the vagaries and caprices of the gods. Unreasonable as it is today, it is still quite interesting, philosophically and anthropologically speaking.

So, here comes Hippocrates, who reasonably argued that disease was not a form of punishment inflicted to humans by gods, but rather the consequence of a combination of environmental factors, such as a person's everyday diet and their living habits. Indeed, you can search all you want — you will not find a single mention of the mystical element concerning diseases in the entirety of the Hippocratic Corpus (*Corpus Hippocratum*), the one used to draw up the Hippocratic oath). His absolute separation of medicine from religion made his entire study of diseases and their potential cures possible. So, maybe this is what made Hippocrates the quintessential physician; offering cures over prayers. Or maybe it was his attention up to the last detail and his unprecedented professionalism. Then again, maybe it was his ethical standards and high morality values when it came to dealing with patients, no matter the particularities of their situation. Either way,

"WELLNESS": A NEW WORD FOR ANCIENT IDEAS

Hippocrates served as the central figure in ancient Greek medicine, but there were other noteworthy practitioners as well, of course.

Homoeopathists find in the Hippocratic writings the roots of their doctrines. Naturopaths, chiropractors, herbalists, and osteopaths invoke him as the founder of the ideals that underlie their own approaches to health, disease, and healing. Hippocratic medicine is holistic, so the Hippocratic doctor needed to know his patient thoroughly: what his social, economic, and familial circumstances were, how they lived, what they ate and drank, whether they had traveled or not, whether they were a slave or free, and what their tendencies to disease were. Then, they offered advice on diet and other aspects of healthy living.

By the 5th century BC, there were attempts to identify the material causes for illnesses rather than spiritual ones and this led to a move away from superstition towards scientific enquiry, although, in reality, the two would never be wholly separated. Then, Greek medical practitioners began to show a greater interest in the body itself and to explore the connection between cause and effect, the relation of symptoms to the illness itself and the success or failure of various treatments. Medical practitioners before him paved the way for his accomplishments and those after him elaborated upon said accomplishments. The man who founded the Hippocratic school brought a whole new light and level to the field of medicine, saving a reaching-for-the-stars number of lives along the way.

His contributions to the science of medicine include, among other things, detailed observations of diseases and their effects, as well as an innovative understanding of how health is widely influenced by our dietary habits, breakdowns in bodily processes and, of course, the environment. He also described human veins and bloodletting procedures to relieve the pain in several parts of the body. Facts about the life of the historical Hippocrates are unfortunately rare and he and his medical contributions are sufficiently shadowy to allow a multiplicity of interpretations to be hung from him. It is known, however, that he was born on the island of Cos into a family of doctors. He taught at the highly-regarded medical school on the island and traveled extensively throughout not just Ancient Greece but also the Middle East giving lectures on his subject. He was quite famous during his lifetime and he died at a fairly old age (at the estimated age of 83) in the town of Larissa.

The contributions to Ancient Greek medicine of Hippocrates, Socrates, and others had also a lasting influence on Islamic medicine and medieval European medicine until many of their findings eventually became obsolete in the 14th century. The earliest known Greek medical school opened in Cnidus in 700 BC. Alcmaeon, author of the first anatomical compilation, worked at this school, and it was here that the practice of observing patients was established. Despite their respect for Egyptian medicine, attempts to discern any particular influence on Greek practice at this early time had not been dramatically successful, because of the lack of sources and the challenge of understanding ancient medical terminology. It is clear, however, that the Greeks imported Egyptian substances into their pharmacopoeia, and the influence became more pronounced after the establishment of a school of Greek medicine in Alexandria, Egypt.

As previously mentioned, Hippocrates was the founder of a new school where he tried to clearly separate medical knowledge from the various myths and (either religious or not) superstitions of his era. His *Corpus Hippocratum* is the main source of modern knowledge for his methods and discoveries. It is a collection of 70 volumes that had been gathered in the great Library of Alexandria around 200 BC. These volumes are an ocean of medical material, touching lots of different medical sectors (such as anatomy, pathology, etc.), and probably they were not written by Hippocrates alone. It is estimated that only few of those books were written by him, however all of them are considered to be an expression of his medical teachings and philosophy.

In Hippocratic medicine, effective treatment relied on examining the patient holistically. Diet, sleep, work and exercise were all seen as important factors that could play a role in producing and reversing the imbalance in humors that was believed to result in illness. Hippocratic medicine was based on the natural philosophy the Greeks had been developing since the 500s BC. It used careful observation, logical deduction, experimentation and record-keeping. Hippocratic doctors

"WELLNESS": A NEW WORD FOR ANCIENT IDEAS

were cautious and skeptical, a view summed up by their famous saying: 'The art is long; life is short; the occasion fleeting; experience fallacious, and judgment difficult.'

This great personality is also credited of being one of the very first to write about preventive medicine. More precisely, he and his followers were very concerned about preserving their health through proper diet and activities, such as exercise and getting enough rest in relation to their manual work. Hippocrates was not content to simply study the causes and the treatments of each disease. He advised medical practitioners to be responsible and serious about their profession and have high moral standards. All doctors still swear to his aforementioned oath where these standards are embodied. Hippocrates' approach to healing and the role of the doctor has been influencing international and western in particular medicine ever since.

According to him, medical practitioners should be clean and neat, serious, honest, understanding, and trustworthy. They should have a clean workspace and all the necessary instruments for their work, and follow through precise techniques for bandaging, splinting and so on. He even goes so far as to dictate the proper maintenance of fingernails. This detailed manner of professionalism, discipline and rigorous practice is one of his lasting prescriptions that forever changed the face of the medical industry globally and in an unprecedented way.

Hippocrates, and his followers, were the first to accurately describe and analyze some medical conditions. This included determining the clubbing of fingers, sometimes referred to as "Hippocratic fingers", as an important diagnostic sign in chronic suppurative lung disease, lung cancer and cyanotic heart disease. His methods for treating hemorrhoids, in addition, are still used today, though, thankfully, with more sophisticated instruments. Finally, parts of his work in pulmonary medicine and surgery have not been improved upon since Ancient Greece. Hippocrates was the first documented chest surgeon and his techniques, while crude, such as the use of lead pipes to drain chest wall abscess, are still valid. Moreover, the Hippocratic School imbued physicians with the significance of making meticulous observations and keeping clinical documentation. Hippocrates himself probably kept careful and extensive notes of his patients' symptoms, including pulse, fever, complexion, pains and excretions. He went on to include family history and environment in order to have a full, comprehensive understanding of each individual's situation.

Hippocrates' school of thought put prognosis first while diagnosis followed. This is kind of defective by nature since it means that medical practitioners predicted outcomes based primarily on statistical data and information about the patient, rather than locating the exact source of the problem by examining the sick individual. Hippocratic philosophy focused on taking care of the patient by using nature's unique and undeniable healing powers. It was truly believed that nature, and not medical practitioners, was the one to do most of the healing. Therefore, doctors should not get in nature's way, but rather facilitate, if not accelerate, the recovery process with proper nutrition, meticulous cleanliness, and always sufficient rest.

This was fairly successful at the time and in accordance with the medical philosophy of the phrase "primum non nocerum" which means "first, do no harm." It can be demonstrated with the example of a broken bone in an arm or a leg. Instead of interfering with that bone's natural ability to restore itself to its original condition, the medical practitioner should set up the necessary brace or splint to help the patient remain immobile. Of course, such a passive treatment method was only effective for relatively simple ailments and so it was the easy target of serious criticism over the next centuries from more modern physicians. For example, the French physician M.S. Houdart called that Hippocratic method a "meditation upon death".

In his book, "On Airs, Waters, and Places," Hippocrates stresses that environmental conditions help shape not only the character and the creativity of a people, but their very health as well. The various diseases that may plague them result from the place's microclimate, their dietary habits, the quality of the potable water et cetera.

Hippocrates was also the first to combine scientific observation with experiment and philosophy. He fought popularly established superstitions and used common sense as his base for philosophically defining humans and the world. He was a seeker of harmony, in the human body, in the human soul, and in nature as well. The fundamental principles of the Hippocratic approach are easily discernible in both Holistic and Homeopathic Medicine.

Hippocrates was based on the properties of fire and water to explain of what humans and nature consisted. He believed that disease prevention is based upon maintaining the balance between liquid substances, heat, cold and drought, which he associated with the four humors of the human body – a theory that we will discuss extensively later on, because it is of utmost importance in the chapter of Ancient Greek medical history. According to Hippocrates, a physician has to restore the balance between those four liquid human humors in order to facilitate nature's therapeutic action. He used many plants and herbs, because he believed deeply in their powers. Out of the approximately 256 plants he used, many still constitute the base in the production of modern medicines.

What Is Naturopathy?

Naturopathy is the modern-day Hippocratic Therapeutic Science. Hippocrates is credited to have said that "Natural forces within us are the true healers of disease." The science of naturopathy is taught in many countries around the world, mainly in Europe and the US, but unfortunately not in Greece. It is an integrated alternative science focusing not only on the symptomatology of a disease but also on its deeper causes. Its basic principle is that treatment and health restoration are a biological process, like digestion, like the rebuilding of a broken bone or the healing of a wound.

Per naturopathy, the human body has its own wise, innate physiological self-healing system. If that system falls short of doing its work, the choices of the ill individual are to blame; the individual is the one who does not maintain their body right, but rather mishandles what they have to do. A naturopathic can often detect a predisposition of the body before the disease develops. Naturopathy has a natural, drugfree, and operation-free approach towards health. It focuses on three things: finding the cause of the disease, reinforcing the ability of the body to heal itself and improving the lifestyle of the individual. It supports and applies the Hippocratic unifying principle of disease, diagnosis and treatment, that is, that there is but one disease, toxemia. This poisoning of the body results from people's lifestyle usually combined with psychological stress.

Naturopathy does not suppress the symptomatology but rather helps the symptoms complete their work which is to purify the poisoned body. It kind of lets the disease heal itself. Modern science has proven that environmental conditions help define the expression of the genes to a high degree. Genetic expression depends on and is determined by the presence of enzymes that the body itself can produce, depending on the messages it receives; those messages can be biochemical, psychological or natural. Hippocrates said that the symptoms expressed are not the disease, but rather the means that our body uses to defend itself against the disease. For instance, if someone gets poisoned, vomit and diarrhea are the results, the symptoms that the body will use to heal the poisoning.

Naturopathy uses many different means and methods. Its cornerstone is diet. But those dietary changes must be permanent and not occasional. Your naturopathic might prescribe you a few orthomolecular food supplements that will compensate for what modern food lacks because of chemical fertilizers and hybrid varieties. Herbal medicine, massage, Bach flower remedies (BFRs), myoskeletal therapy, homeopathy, and acupuncture are some usual methods of naturopathy. One technique that might need further explanation is iridology aka iridodiagnosis. Iridology is an alternative medicine technique in which patterns, colors, and other characteristics of the patient's iris are examined to determine information about their systemic health. Another one would be auriculotherapy (aka auricular therapy), that is, the stimulation of the auricle of the external ear for the diagnosis and treatment of health conditions in other parts of the body.

"WELLNESS": A NEW WORD FOR ANCIENT IDEAS

The Always Present Herbal Medicine

The use of herbs was expanded in the entire ancient world and Ancient Greece was evidently no exception. Greek physicians used wine, opium, and henbane to help with pain and toothache, and they applied aloe (originally from Egypt) to cure burns. In addition, they used crushed garlic to disinfect cuts, and mint tea to help with stomachaches. And now, you know that a list of the most important plants and herbs will follow, not just because I find this part incredibly interesting but also because I am a plant lover. In previous studies, I have talked about my love for animals; in this one, I have the chance to reveal my love for the extraordinarily rich flora of our planet.

In the country of Greece, one can find 40% of Europe's medicinal plants. And yet, it pains me to say that we do not produce (nor export, obviously) any herbal preparation. The only relative production has to do with aromatic plants, but it is only small-scale (0.05% of the country's cultivable surface). Greece has 700 medicinal plants, but does not use its great development potential. A big multinational enterprise has financed multiple researches on Homer's *Odyssey* texts that talk about herbal preparations, while experiments are conducted in India in order to ascertain which medicines described by Hippocrates can still be utilized today. Homer talks about androphores, that is poisonous herbs, painkilling medicines, and medicines that were damaging for the psyche. In *Odyssey*, an herb called nepenthes is mentioned, which is thought to be a sedative and to quell all sorrows with forgetfulness; it probably caused an increase in serotonin.

So, let's start off with **spearmint**, which was then used as a vaginal cleansing and now it is recommended, in the form of an infusion, for nausea, dyspepsia, migraine, colic, fever, spasms, cramps, and gallstones. It has antispasmoic, sweating, alleviating, sedative and digestive effects. As a poultice, it relieves from rheumatisms and neuralgias. It can also help fight certain skin diseases and reduce the swelling of the breasts during the breast-feeding period.

According to the writings of Hippocrates, **laurel** was used to ease women's pregnancy. Nowadays, it is used in the form of herb tea to help deal with intestinal disorders. Laurel's essential oil is considered to be a very strong analgesic and antiseptic.

Fennel in Ancient Greece was used for vaginal pains and metrorrhagia. Today, it is considered to protect from eye ache, cystitis, arthritis, asthma, and an upset stomach. Marjoram was used as a laxative; now it is indicated for the treatment of muscular pain, sprained ankles, and neuralgias.

Sage was recommended for pulmonary diseases and as a vaginal analgesic. Today, sage infusion works as a diuretic and as a detoxifying agent and is recommended for those suffering from arthritis. It helps in laryngitis, and it stimulates the digestive and nervous systems. Compresses with sage can alleviate the pain from cuts and wounds, while washing with sage oil is considered to fight dandruff.

Women used **myrtle** to wash their sensitive area, while the extracts of its boiled leaves were thought to relieve their pain during pregnancy. Now, myrtle is recommended in cases of toothache, for treating inflammations and infections of the gastrointestinal system, while its essential oil has antiseptic properties.

Wild rose was used in Ancient Greece in the form of poultice for edemas and inflammations. In the present time, the infusion of its petals is used as a diuretic agent and as a nerve palliative. It is also beneficial for combatting insomnia, constipation, and chronic enteritis. The infusion made from the wild rose leaves works as a medicine for diarrhea and kidney stones. Its fruits are considered to be diuretics, refreshing, and rich in vitamins. Lastly, the concoction made from its petals is stimulant and cleansing.

In addition, ancient Greek medicine recognized that various herbs contributed differently to the body's wellness as they had particular affinities to certain organs, tissues or parts of the body. Herbs whose action focuses on the heart are called cordials; herbs that treat conditions of the head are called cephalics; liver tonics are called hepatics; finally, digestive tonics are called stomachics, and so on. Like other traditional systems of herbal medicine, Greek physicians used the principles of herbal taste and energetics to further refine their therapeutic classification and herbs usage. For instance, herbs

"WELLNESS": A NEW WORD FOR ANCIENT IDEAS

for the stomach that are cooling and detoxifying are called bitter stomachics. These are indicated for hot, inflammatory, hyper-acidic or bilious stomach conditions. Aromatic stomachics gently harmonize and stimulate gastric function in cases of inactivity and stomach congestion. Pungent stomachics are even hotter and more stimulating and they remove excess cold and phlegm pretty effectively. Out of all the herbs that relieve pain, the ones called anodynes are those who can relax and disperse muscular pains in the most effective way through their gentle warming and dispersing action.

In herbal prescribing, it is also necessary to adjust the prescribed formula to the constitutional nature of the patient. For example, those with a stronger constitution will be better able to withstand the rigors of radical purgatives, whereas those with a more delicate constitution will require a more moderate and gradual cleansing. Additionally, factors, such as the weather, the climate, and all environmental conditions must be taken into account when prescribing herbal medicines. For instance, if the weather is cold, a formula to warm the body and fight chills must be more heating in nature than if those chills were caught in relatively warm weather.

What's more, in ancient Greek medicine, several different innovative and efficient herbal preparations, designed to deliver maximum healing power to the part of the body with the disorder, were used in treatment. Herbal teas, pills, or powders were mixed and matched with various standard preparations, like syrups or tinctures, which were kept on hand. External or topical treatment methods, such as compresses, liniments, salves, poultices or cataplasms, and fomentations were equally used.

The practical details of Ancient Greek medical system of herbal healing arose from the accumulated clinical experience of many generations of Greek physicians.

Move Your Body

I have already said much about medicine in Ancient Greece and have not talked about physical exercise which was a key factor to the maintaining of good health; something that many modern Hollywood movies have made widely known worldwide. Well, yes, the ancient Greeks believed that mental and physical health were closely related as they had found that the body and mind should be in harmony.

It was all about balance and harmony. Aristotle believed that sports and gymnastics were fundamental to the development of the human body to optimize functional capacity, physical wellbeing and harmony between mind and body, hence the famous phrase *"healthy mind in a healthy body"* which is still widely used in Greece.

In fact, it has been proven that exercise of moderate intensity may serve to improve attention and scholastic performance. In Ancient Greece, physical activity was a necessary part of the training done in schools, primarily to promote physical and mental health. Health promotion appeared during the Olympic Games since the care of athletes and prevention of injuries were specialist services provided by instructors called "paidotrivai".

According to Hippocrates's study *"On Food,"* for the exercises that were done by athletes, olive oil was used to increase body temperature, to help the warming up and for muscles to be flexible so as to avoid sport injuries. Also, figs and other fruits with high glucose concentration that provide energy were offered to athletes to improve their performance.

The Father of Medicine – Part II

Hippocrates – each time I type that name, it gives me goosebumps – was astonishingly explicit concerning what to do and what to use for every single ailment or disease discovered. For instance, in case of side pains, either the patient or a physician should dip a large soft sponge in water and apply gently. If the pain reached the collarbone, then making the elbow bleed was recommended until the flowing blood becomes bright red. In case of pneumonia, a physician should give the patient a bath to relieve the pain and help the patient bring up phlegm. During the bath, the patient must remain completely still. For chest diseases, Hippocrates mentioned that barley soup with vinegar and honey would bring up phlegm that needed to get out of the patient's system.

Furthermore, the first classification of mental disorders proposed by Hippocrates was: mania, melancholy, phrenitis, insanity, disobedience, paranoia, panic, epilepsy, and hysteria. Some of these terms are still used today. Psychological and mental illnesses were viewed as a nature's effect on people and thus were treated like other diseases. Hippocrates argued that the brain is the organ responsible for mental illnesses and that intelligence and sensitivity reach the brain through the mouth, through the breath. He believed that mental illnesses can be treated more effectively if they are handled in a similar manner to physical medical conditions. According to Hippocrates, the diagnosis and treatment of mental and physical diseases must be based on observation, on consideration of the causes, and on the balance and the four humors theories.

As I implicitly said in the beginning, Hippocrates developed the four humors theory. But let's take things from the start. First of all, humourism, aka humoralism, was a system of medicine detailing the makeup and workings of the human body, adopted by the Indian Ayurveda system of medicine, and Ancient Greek and Roman physicians and philosophers, positing that an excess or deficiency of any of four distinct bodily fluids in a person – the humors – directly influences their temperament and health.

The humoralist system of medicine was highly individualistic, seeing that, according to its theory, each individual patient was said to have their own unique humoral composition. Moreover, it resembled a holistic approach to medicine as the link between mental and physical processes were emphasized by this framework. From Hippocrates onward, the humoral theory was adopted by Greek, Roman and Islamic physicians, and became the most commonly held view of the human body among European physicians until the advent of modern medical research in the 19th century. The concept has not been used in medicine since then.

The four humors of Hippocratic medicine are black bile, yellow bile, phlegm, and blood. Each of them corresponds to one of the four temperaments of the traditional theory. According to the "four temperaments" theory, there are four fundamental personality types. This proto-psychological theory's types are: sanguine (optimistic and social), choleric (short-tempered and irritable), melancholic (analytical and quiet), and phlegmatic (relaxed and peaceful). Most formulations include the possibility of various mixtures of these four personality types.

It was Hippocrates who incorporated the four temperaments into his medical theories as part of the ancient medical concept of humourism, arguing that four bodily fluids affect human personality traits and behaviors. In accordance with that concept, doctors would try to balance out the four humors to cure their patients. More precisely, they kept their patients warm when they had a cold, they kept patients with fever and sweat cool and dry, they made patients bleed if there was the need for blood balance restoration, and they "purged" patients to restore their bile balance. This would be attained by giving them laxatives or diuretics, or by making them vomit.

The first two treatment methods still make sense in modern science, the third one does not, while the fourth one is not a generally applied rule; it all depends on the individual's illness. For example, if the patient has eaten or swallowed by mistake something toxic, inducing vomiting might be the right way to go. Another example results from their belief that if an individual had too much blood, that would give them a fever. So, the appropriate medical treatment would be reducing the amount of blood in the body. Greek physicians did that by cutting the patient's arm a little until enough blood had run out; this was supposed to bring down the patient's fever. Another choice in the case of fever would be putting leeches on the patient's arm to suck the redundant amount of blood out. Later discoveries in biochemistry have lead modern medical science to reject the theory of the four temperaments, even though some personality type systems of varying scientific acceptance continue to use four or more categories of a similar nature.

Moreover, Hippocrates realized that the movement — at least, partially — of all bodily organs is downward. He related them to the function of the digestive tube, because the digestive tube's end is indeed the anal orifice. Through inhalation and the consequent downward movement (depression) of the diaphragm, the lungs follow a downward route and, this way, they serve the downward movement of the digestive tube. Through the diaphragm depression, the lungs knead the content of the stomach and push the content of the intestines downwards. Concerning the lungs' movement, this thought is predominant in TCM. Through the production and circulation of the bile, which flows into the digestive tube through the biliary system, the liver promotes the intestine's downward movement. Through the urine production and circulation, the latter also being downward through the urethra, the kidneys also participate in the downward movement of the third pair of Meridians. This pair's chiasm at the area of the shoulder-blades reveals the high level of understanding and knowledge that Hippocrates had about the human body's function. It equally reveals an understanding of the communication and balance between the right and left sides of the body which led Hippocrates to the conclusion that we can treat the right side for problems of the left. Finally, the chiasm of the third Meridian pair shows that Hippocrates realized there is a change in the energy polarity throughout the transition from the exterior part of the body (temple, nape) to the interior (lungs, liver, kidneys, spleen, mammary gland). This 'chiasm' idea exists in TCM (Hand Yang Ming chiasm at the upper lip of the mouth, Yin Qiao Mai chiasm inside the skull) as well as in modern Western medicine (the chiastic pyramid structure).

Hippocrates knew and taught a therapeutic technique he called 'phlebotomy' (vein incision). This technique perfectly corresponds to acupuncture both in theory and in practice. At this point, we have to talk about those terms because they might be a little confusing. When Hippocrates uses the term "vein," he is talking about vascular stems that host the flow of venous blood. These canals are not the ones we call "veins" today. The canals that Hippocrates described sometimes move on the surface and sometimes inside the body and one can intervene by applying the so-called phlebotomy.

It is totally normal that this therapeutic technique was forgotten over time, considering the persecutions that followed everything that was Greek from the Roman times until today. Many pieces of Ancient Greek knowledge sank into oblivion. On the contrary, the Chinese kept their ancient healing arts through time; it is the nature of their culture that makes them keep their memory that way.

Let's Go Meet a Few More Notable Personalities (and Their Contribution to Medicine)

Greek physicians also believed that some kinds of climate tended to increase the amount of certain humors in the body. If someone lived in a wet, cold climate, that would tend to increase their amount of phlegm, for instance. Thus, one treatment might be to move to a drier, warmer climate to balance out the four humors again. Yes, this was another one of the wrongly believed ideas.

Galen of Pergamon introduced a system of four degrees for each of the four basic conditions to measure more precisely how hot, cold, wet or dry an herb is. This allowed physicians and pharmacists to formulate and prescribe medicines with more accuracy. Accuracy is critical in herbal medicine, since the usual method of herbal treatment is to use medicines whose nature is either opposed or complementary to the nature of the disorder and, at the same time, the herbal medicine had to be equal to the imbalance by degree with the aim to bring balance back into the patient's body. Galen was a prominent Greek physician, surgeon, and philosopher in the Roman Empire. Arguably the most accomplished of all medical researchers of antiquity, he influenced the progress of numerous scientific sectors, including anatomy, physiology, pathology, pharmacology, and neurology, as well as philosophy and logic.

The temperament theory has its roots in the ancient four humors theory. It may originate from Ancient Egypt or Mesopotamia, but

"WELLNESS": A NEW WORD FOR ANCIENT IDEAS

it was the Greek physician Hippocrates who developed it into a medical theory. The four humors theory, though fundamentally flawed, established the notion of physical causes for illness, and provided a foundation for the practice of diagnosis and treatment. For example, if a patient felt lethargic, a practitioner of the Hippocratic method would diagnose an overabundance of phlegm, and then prescribe citrus as a treatment.

Despite the flaws of the humoral theory, Hippocrates kept an open enough mind and, in his writings, he warned against the dangers of letting theory jump too far ahead of the clinical practice and anything that can actually produce tangible medical results. To stress that necessity of tradition and a practical approach, he said: "Foolish the doctor who despises knowledge acquired by the ancients."

Aristotle (384-322 BC) was definitely one of the greatest contributors to Ancient Greek medicine, after Hippocrates. What he did was study the work of the latter while using his own skills of deduction. This inevitably led to some crucial misunderstandings, the most famous one being Aristotle's belief that the human body was controlled by the heart and not the brain. His most remarkable contribution to medicine was his teleological understanding of disease. According to this point of view, symptoms appear as the observable effect of some physical cause. From this elementary understanding, Aristotle applied scientific practices, such as critical observation and logic, in his own development of treatments. He also advocated the practice of dissection to understand physical processes.

Together with Plato (423-347 BC), Aristotle came to the conclusion that the human body had no use in the afterlife. This new way of thinking was spread around and influenced Greek physicians, who in Alexandria, Egypt, started dissecting dead bodies and studying them. Sometimes, even the bodies of alive criminals were cut open. It was through this kind of research that Herophilus (335-280 BC) came to the opposite conclusion of that of Aristotle. Herophilus understood that it was the brain that controlled the movement of limbs and not the heart. Aristotle's and Plato's philosophies, writings and speeches allowed the Greeks to begin to find out about the inside of the human body in a systematic way. The great minds of the era pushed science forward, so that medical professionals, scientists and researchers could seek out entirely natural theories for the cause of diseases.

Alcmaeon of Croton (circa 500 BC) is regarded as one of the most eminent medical theorists and philosophers in ancient history. It is believed that he was a student of Pythagoras. He wrote widely on medicine; however, some historians say he was probably more of a philosopher of science, rather than a physician. As far as we know, he was the first one to wonder about the possible internal causes of illnesses. He put forward the idea that an illness may be caused by environmental problems, nutrition and lifestyle.

Pythagoras was born around 580 BC and, by advocating a vegetarian diet, he established another revelatory connection between an individual's diet and health. Alcmaeon, who lived in the 5th century BC, was the one to discover the optic nerve. Now, the most renowned physician before Hippocrates, that is Demokedes of Croton, had a public clinic in the city of Athens. His accomplishments included, among other things, the successful treatment of sprained ankles and the removal of tumors.

Thucydides (circa 460-395 BC), a Greek historian, often called the "Father of Scientific History," came to the conclusion that prayers were totally ineffective against diseases. He added that epilepsy could be scientifically explained and that it had nothing to do with angry gods or evil spirits. Erasistratus (304-250 BC) was the one to find out that blood moves through the veins. However, he overlooked the fact that it circulates.

The methods that were used in Ancient Greece for reaching to a diagnosis were not that different, as one would expect, from the ones used in modern times. Many of their natural remedies are similar to effective home-made remedies still used. Their theory of the four humors, though, was basically an obstacle to the progress of the medical sector – about 2,000 years later, it was found to be a false one. Physicians used to carry out a clinical observation at first; they performed a thorough physical examination of the patient. They would

"WELLNESS": A NEW WORD FOR ANCIENT IDEAS

often refer to the Hippocratic body of work for guidance on how to carry it out and which diseases they should consider or try to rule out.

Even though religion was slowly but steadily making way to logical reasoning, people still asked of their (many) gods to heal them at the Asclepeion, in Epidaurus, and other sacred temples. Despite the apparent period of enlightenment, even doctors — not just the patients — would still appeal to the gods if the treatment they used was not as effective as they hoped it would be. Some doctors would treat their patients and then take them to the abaton and let them sleep there; the abaton was the holiest part of a temple. They believed that Hygeia (health) and Panacea, daughters of Asclepius would arrive with their two holy snakes that would cure the patients. The snake today is the symbol of pharmacists. On a side note, the term "hygiene" is derived from the word *hygeia*.

Of course, temples like that eventually became health spas, gymnasiums, public baths, and sports stadiums. And over time, magic and calling out to the gods gave way to looking for the natural causes of all diseases. This step was what led to the research for natural cures and remedies. So, Ancient Greek physicians became herbal plants experts and began prescribing natural remedies. They were convinced that nature is the mightiest healer.

Hypnosis

In Ancient Greek mythology, Hypnos (meaning "sleep" — you might have guessed it thanks to the term "hypnosis") was personified. I would like to implicitly give you his very interesting family tree and then we will get right away to the concept of hypnosis and the methods used in Ancient Greece. Hypnos's mother was Nyx, the deity of Night, and his father was Erebus, the deity of Darkness. As for his children, they were the gods of dreams: Morpheus (shape), Phobetor (fear), and Phantasos (imagination). So, in the Darkness of the Night, people's Fears and Imagination get entwined, take Shape, and we see the result in our Sleep. Pretty mystical — *and* genius — If you ask me.

As previously noted, hypnosis derives from the Greek mythological personification of sleep – his Roman equivalent is known as Somnus (as in somnolence, somnambulist, and many more). Somnus lived in a cave where the rays of the sun could not enter and there were plants with hypnotic properties at its entrance. Ancient Greeks considered sleep to be a very important state for two main reasons. Firstly, because of its therapeutic effects and also because of the value and the power Greeks gave to dreams. The relation between sleep and therapy is mostly due to Asclepius's therapeutic worship and the practices of this worship, something that continued to exist during the "more scientific" period of Hippocratic Medicine. In fact, Hippocrates himself said that both states of being asleep and of being vigilant can be detrimental when practiced in excessive quantities. He also thought that diseases to which sleep caused dysphoria (discomfort) were deadly, while diseases to which sleep was beneficial were not deadly.

However, apart from the teachings of Hippocrates, who placed sleep in a wider scope of therapeutic activities, sleep also occupied the very center of a specific therapeutic practice associated with the worship of Asclepius. Therapeutic hypnosis was practiced in the Asclepeions. These were healing and therapeutic temples, consecrated to Asclepius, the Greek God of Medicine; they were basically the first hospitals, which is by itself of particular interest. They operated throughout the dominion of Ancient Greece from the Bronze Age until the 6th century AD. They were approximately 300 and they covered the territory from Southern Italy and Sicily all the way to Minor Asia, the most important ones being located in Epidaurus, Cos, Bergama, and Athens.

Hypnosis was a ceremonial practice, a ritual, the climax of a particular process. In Ancient Greece, people used to sleep in holy places, such as temples, with the aim to have (to "receive") a revealing dream for either oracular or therapeutic reasons. For the Assyrians, the Babylonians and the Egyptians, in the Serapeum (temple consecrated to Serapis) and the Iseum (temple consecrated to Isis), that ceremonial decubitus was mostly associated with oneiromancy (divination) and necromancy (divination involving the dead), while in Minor Asia, it was

"WELLNESS": A NEW WORD FOR ANCIENT IDEAS

the priests that performed said ritual for the faithful. In Ancient Greece, hypnosis was inextricably linked with pre-Hippocratic Medicine, that is the therapeutic approach applied in the aforementioned healing temples consecrated to Asclepius. So, hypnosis was mostly associated with Asclepius' Holy Medicine and reflected more widely how the concept of cure and therapy was perceived in Ancient Greece.

Following a process of catharsis in both body and soul, the patient-supplicant then went to sleep in a holy place, seeking for an apocalyptic therapy dream, a divine meeting within the dream, which will mark their cure. The priests who followed the faithful believers had to create a strong feeling of self-suggestion and religious elevation so that God would appear in their dream, while reverent hymns were chanted. The preparations included special diets, fasting, baths, watching theatrical and musical shows, reading, physical exercise, massage, inhaling fumes (possibly by using psychotropic substances) and discussing with the priests and physicians of the Asclepeion.

The use of running water was fundamental in hypnosis, while the patients also drank tea made from various herbs and other therapeutic mixtures with sedative properties and sometimes they were already cured at this point. The substances used were only known by the priests and, as I said before, it is possible that they were psychotropic. It is probable that, afterwards, the priests examined the bowels of the sacrificed animals to give the green light for the continuation of the process, with hypnosis functioning as the means for the individual's therapy. The "therapeutic" dream was the climax of the entire process.

Asclepius appeared in those dreams as a bearded man holding his Rod (aka his Staff aka the asklepian), a serpent-entwined rod, or as a male hand touching the affected part of the patient's body. Therapeutic dreams with snakes in them were also frequent. A good sign of therapy was also the appearance of a dog – as Asclepius had a dog as a friend – and equally that of a rooster, which was another symbol of the God of Medicine. The following day, the patients described to the priests what they saw in their dream and, depending on the content of the dream, they got the corresponding treatment, if they were not already cured.

We can easily understand that hypnosis, by nature, had some characteristics of initiation, so priests and healers were required to have special knowledge. On the other hand, there appeared to be no social discrimination; everyone was entitled to seek for their cure – the rich and the poor, the kings and the plebeians. Only the moribund and pregnant women were not allowed. Hypnosis also had some ceremonial and mystical features and, despite its advantages and good results, it was opposed to the new perception of medicine, introduced and brought forward by Hippocrates, who always searched for a rational approach to handling diseases and ailments. He refused to accept divine intervention as the cause of diseases; he did not negate Asclepius or anything, of course, but he placed him in a greater distance from people and nature. He perceived health and sickness as natural phenomena that had to be understood and dealt with as everyday facts in human life.

The practice of hypnosis, that is the apocalyptic-therapeutic dream, is all but lost. Many medicines, treatments, beliefs, plant uses and other things we saw and will see later on in this study are still used or practiced today; hypnosis is undoubtedly one of them. I bet you all know someone in your family or from your friends who still believes – passionately, but not admittedly – in future-telling dreams and who wants to know their meaning as soon as possible. Hypnosis has survived remarkably in the Christian Era until today as a popular tradition for predicting the future. It is part of the concept of holistic medicine, which recognizes that every biochemical and neurophysiological function is inextricably linked to human psyche, and that spiritual and mental elevation is an indispensable therapeutic process. The diagnostic and therapeutic aspects of dreams are now an integral part of the psychotherapeutic concept. Practices, such as dream incubation, dream therapy, hyper-personal psychotherapy, and hypnotherapy, constitute an attempt of reconnection with the ancient, holy medicine of Asclepius.

"WELLNESS": A NEW WORD FOR ANCIENT IDEAS

Melampus, the First Psychiatrist

The first psychiatrist, who was also an oracle, a seer, is said to be from Greece; more precisely, from Argos. His name was Melampus. He was a fourth-generation descendant of Deucalion and the ethnarch of the clairvoyant Melampodides clan. Melampus was a prominent figure in Ancient Greek mythology and was praised notably in antiquity. Among several other women from Argos, he managed to cure the daughters of the King of Argos, Proetus, from a disease that was called "mania." And among other things, he used *Helleborus niger* (aka Christmas rose, aka black hellebore) in his treatment methods for the act of purifying. Plinius mentions another (similar) version of events: that Melampus gave the women from Argos to drink milk from goats who had eaten hellebore.

Thanks to that success, he became one of the three Kings of Argos and his mythical treatment method for mania with black hellebore conquered for more than 3,000 years both the popular and scientific medicines. This is actually an impressive feat, considering that modern-day experiments on psychopathic individuals use hellebore as well, even if the results are mostly negative. The academics Georgios Tsoukantas and D. Kouretis, who were based on the meticulous study of ancient texts and preserved art masterpieces from the 5th century BC, revealed that certain modern discoveries were actually already known by our ancestors in antiquity. According to said academics, the myth that accompanies Melampus and the way he became an oracle refers in reality to treatments of diseases of psychogenic etiology in the 14th century BC.

Apart from the pharmacological aspect of the subject, Melampus and his treatment method for mania offered another great subject to later research: the position that the ancient medico-oracle in the ancient people's conscience and his influence in the History of Medicine. It is equally important that Ancient Greek doctors of 1,400 BC had a knowledge of psychotherapy, group therapy, psychosomatic therapy and also psychanalysis. Pythagoras, in particular, stressed the value of group psychotherapy, medical herbs and music for the treatment of emotionally ill patients.

Mental Health Issues

A great number of scientists and writers has addressed the subject of mania. The ancient thought accepts that all types of mental disorder are the result of supernatural intervention. Herodotus recognized at least two types of mania: one type that is maleficent and of supernatural origin and another one that is due to natural causes. Empedocles had separated the ex *purgamento animae* mania from the type of mania that is due to a physical disease. Of course, the ancient layman considered any sort of mania to be a supernatural force that was inflicted upon people as punishment.

At the Classical Era, people used to avoid the mentally ill, because they were individuals carrying a divine curse. Any contact with them involved danger; they threw rocks at them to keep them at bay or took other protective measures. On the other hand, they did show them a great respect and sometimes they were in awe in front of them because of their ability to get in touch with the supernatural world and at times they could show powers that were forbidden to the ordinary people, or as we usually call them in Greek: the "common mortals."

Hippocrates' book *On the Sacred Disease* in his body of work *Corpus Hippocraticum* deals with the matter and is the most characteristic sample concerning the way of thinking and the dealing with those sacred seizures. Hippocrates' work, as well as oracles, rejected Melampus' medical use of hellebore. Medico-oracles had an important place in antiquity because they fulfilled people's need for treatment. However, the difference between medical and ritualistic purification started to show, no matter their similar purifying ideal (a natural one and a supernatural one, respectively). The medical-natural was necessary for life and health and the ritualistic-supernatural was necessary for people's relationship with gods and the divine element.

Finally, I would like to stay a little more on the subject of treating mental illnesses because, in 2007, excavations began in the ancient Greek city Vathoneia (located just outside Istanbul) lead by the substitute professor Şengül Aydıngün of the Koçaeli Universitesi. According to him, the 700 recipients found constitute an important and

"WELLNESS": A NEW WORD FOR ANCIENT IDEAS

unique discovery since it was only the first time that such an amount of findings came to light in one single archaeological excavation project. The findings included hundreds of ceramic and glass little pots like bottles containing traces of antidepressants and medicines for the heart. They also included mortars of various sizes, powders, and an ancient type of stove. Therefore, there was probably a medicine production center in the area, where medicinal plants were also cultivated since 7000 BC. The findings also prove that Istanbul – then Constantinople – was sieged in 626 AD by a united force of Avars and the Sassanid Persians, but this is hardly our study's concern.

I must also mention that there was this concept, "physis," which was first proposed by none other than Hippocrates. We already saw that he changed – or evolved, some might argue – hieratic or theocratic medicine into a rational discipline. The basic structure of the Asclepeion in Cos points to the fact that Hippocrates believed in a holistic healthcare model, and in his school science met with drug therapy, diet, and physical and mental exercise, as well as divine solicitation. Furthermore, the Asclepeion of Cos offered all patients general treatment that included physical exercise, massage and walks considered necessary to restore health, well-being of the soul and the inner peace of man, and using dreams both for diagnostic and for therapeutic reasons. To achieve the desired therapeutic result, the therapist should have prior understanding of the concept of soul and its distinction from the body according to the Platonic trisection of the soul.

Other practices that were used in the treatment of physical and mental illnesses were music and theatre. Their role, along with an effort to improve human behavior, was essential. It was believed that healing the soul through music also helped heal the body, and there were actually specific musical applications for certain diseases. For instance, the alternating sound of flute and harp served as a treatment for gout. Asclepius was the first to apply music as a therapy to conquer "passion". Aristotle claims that for some people, the effect of religious melodies that thrill the soul resembles cases of people who have undergone medical treatment and mental catharsis. The ancient tragedies functioned as a form of psychotherapy for patients.

The Theater of Epidaurus at the Ancient Temple of Epidaurus was the place where catharsis took place and where emotions were released through performance. Moreover, "quiet rooms" were designed in which patients would go to sleep so that they could dream of being mentally healthy, and it was believed that this would help them improve their mental health.

EPILOGUE

Let me start off by stating the obvious. Throughout the historical analysis of the medical sector of five countries, we certainly observed many **similarities.** And believe you me, it was pretty hard trying not to repeat the exact same thing over and over. In theory, there were different philosophies for and approaches to medicine, wellness, and health of course, but in practice, we did encounter quite a few similar medical methods and common remedies. This alone does not prove the accuracy of ancient practices, but certainly shows that several different peoples, civilizations, approaches, and philosophies, all ended up functioning under the same beliefs roof.

Despite their differences in approaching a subject, the philosophical basis of all medical schools of thought was the same: the duality (or yin-yang) and the four elements. Secondly, the use of herbs and plants is notably predominant not just in the five countries we studied but around the globe mostly because of the absence of modern-day technology.

Moreover, and more specifically, closely related to the Chinese and Vietnamese traditional medicines are the Japanese and Korean traditional medicines. Historically speaking, many societies in Eastern and Southeastern Asia have been part of the Chinese cultural sphere due to trade, migration, and occupation. Thus, the healing traditions of most Asian cultures are intertwined to some extent, much as their religious philosophies are.

Several accomplishments, mainly medical, that were unknown in the West were known in countries the Muslims conquered. For instance, Muslim doctors were largely based on writings, such as the 12-volumed 'Pathology' by Alexander of Tralles (525 – 605 AD) which includes a detailed description for 120 kinds of surgery, from mastectomy to kidney stones removal surgery, and the '16 Books on Medicine' by Aetius, a gigantic body of work. The 7th volume is on ophthalmology and Muslim doctors actually evolved the cataract removal technique that is described in that volume. Similarly, the great scientist Alhazen is said to have embraced the Aristotelian thought and the Greek rationalism. He believed that the Koran was a fabrication and he considered human thought to be more important than tradition. The notable personalities Avicenna and Rhazes whose contribution we studied were also skeptical concerning religion and were even considered apostates. In modern medicine, TCM is the predominant pole of completion and opposition (Yin – Yang); it gains more and more ground and receives more and more recognition around the world and especially in the West.

As if we did not find enough common ground between the Ancient Greek medicine and TCM along the way, a further analysis of the **numbers**' deepest meaning reveals even more similarities within these two medical systems. The first three numbers (1, 2, 3) express the structure plan of the world. Through the number 4, the first three forces are arranged accordingly to materialize the world. The Chinese attribute the **four primary forces** of the universe to the number 4. The YUEN force expresses the material creation, development, and blooming (Spring), the HENG force expresses the climax form of vegetation and fruition (Summer), the LI force expresses the first downward movement and return to Mother Earth (Fall) and, finally, the ZHI force expresses the introversion and the climax of the downward movement (Winter). In TCM, the 4 primary forces theory has two main characteristics: firstly, that all phenomena have comparable qualities with those 4 forces and that they can be classified on that basis, and, secondly, that within said 4 forces there are internal connections with a controlling (Yin) or creative (Yang) quality. The Ancient Greek medicine follows the Chinese concerning those two characteristics: Heraclitus has described the internal connections between the 4 elements saying that fire lives as earth dies, air lives as fire dies (out), water lives as air dies, and earth lives as water dies.

Concerning **herbology**, one fundamental common element of the two approaches is that each herb is analyzed on two levels. The first level is the analysis of an herb's aspects, that is whether it is wet, dry, warm, cold, astringent or pungent, and whether its taste is sour, bitter, salty or sweet. This first level can be considered as the corresponding to today's biochemical analysis of an herb. The second level is the analysis of an herb's medicinal properties pertaining to various human organs and body parts, using terms such as laxative, diuretic, stimulant, aphrodisiac, softening, vulnerary, emetic, cholagogue, phlegmatic, hematic etc. This analysis is found in both herbal systems, irrespectively of whether they agree on individual herbs.

Of course, there are also certain differences. First of all, the framework of Ancient Greek medicine was largely a **naturalistic** one. Besides, the terms *physician* and *physics* derive from the same Greek root, meaning 'nature'. It is worth mentioning that several different schools of medical thought were developed in Ancient Greece. From the Hippocrates era (5th century BC), those differences already existed. A well-known differentiation was that between the medical school of Knidos, in Minor Asia, and the medical school of Cos. The distinction between those two had to do with the way the human nature functions in the first place and with the way of dealing with disease in the second place. Therefore, we cannot consider Ancient Greek medicine as a single united system; there was also the theory of the triunity of the human soul developed by Plato and the Pythagorean school of thought; and there was also the human soul synthesis developed by Aristotle; however, the school of thought that definitely prevailed was the one developed by Hippocrates.

These phenomena of differentiation and synthesis of ideas that we find in the Ancient Greek medical thought are not equally found neither in the Chinese nor in the modern Western medical thought. In Chinese medicine – traditional or not – there is one fundamental body of work, *The Yellow Emperor's Classic of Internal Medicine*, and everyone and everything is subjected to its writings. One of the reasons why China and Chinese medicine are on the rise is that the people have a deep pragmatism in their behavior. Instead of trying to find somebody to blame when something goes wrong, they ask themselves 'where did I go wrong?' and 'what can I do to make it right?'. So, the distinct personalities in the field of medicine that followed the Yellow Emperor worked to complete his teachings, but certainly not correct or doubt their very founder. We can see the same thing happening within the modern Western medicine. More precisely, there is one central point of view, one main belief and everybody is similarly subjected to it. Nobody questions the idea that microbes and viruses are the cause of an illness. So, there is one well-defined school of medical thought in the Western world, Greece included.

On the other hand, Greece is the country that gave birth to modern medicine through its differentiation and mixture of ideas. So, one single opinion – that of modern technocratic medicine in our case – could not dominate. It is somewhat unavoidable for the predominating model to be questioned and for new schools of medical thought comparable to the Academy of Ancient Greek and Traditional Chinese Medicine to emerge. As usual, only time will tell.

And then, there is **religion**. In antiquity, religion couldn't not play a major role in the way peoples perceived medicine, disease and cure. The monotheism of the Western tradition probably had a deterministic effect on its biomedicine. This distinguished it substantially from the medical systems of the Asian continent. The idea of a single god leads unconsciously to the acceptance of a single truth, a single approach, a single cure for a specific disease or condition. Alternative solutions are seen as heresies, as false beliefs, no matter how popular they may be. On the other hand, the single-mindedness of it all forces one to think in the most logical way in order to reach a conclusion. In biomedicine, existing data within its theory are controlled and processed and the resultant predictions and determinations are almost inescapably based on true facts. And this exactly is the uniqueness of biomedicine from the POV of Asian medical systems.

Apart from religion, another factor that plays an important role in the evolution of **science** is that of the stance of a society's sovereigns. Within Islam, we can see that sciences effloresced during specific periods when knowledge-loving caliphs ruled, like the Abbasids and the Samanids. As a caliphate declines politically with the religious Islamic side taking over, scientific discoveries fall dramatically until they eventually disappear.

I understand that some may be wondering why being preoccupied with the medical practices of the antiquity. Isn't it like dwelling in the past? Hasn't modern medicine already used everything it could use, everything that is of value from the medical knowledge of the (far and near as well) past to evolve? Well, no, it has not. There is always an experiment or a study left to do and, besides, according to archaeologists, there are still discoveries to be made that may fill the numerous gaps of the equally numerous puzzles that the existing discoveries have created.

And this is one of the points I am trying to make with this introductive study: that modern medicine must use **older knowledge** (whether ancient or not) to its full potential because that is the root, the beginning of everything and, as modern discoveries have proven, all the essential medical reality has already been documented in the past. The traditional medicine (or folk medicine) of any country is nowadays unrightfully considered an alternative form of medicine. The standard conventional (industrialized and chemicalized) medicine that has prevailed — as it should; I do not stand for the opposite — is a highly-developed science that uses computerized laboratories, properly sterilized tools and equipment, accurate blood analyses, and industrially produced pills and medicines, among other things. But, haven't we all, at least once, thought of trying to slip back to basics when the going gets tough? When the specialized doctor seems incapable of making it better for us, the so-called 'alternative' solutions are there to give us one last hope that a miracle might still happen, one last chance to smile again. Hopelessness is a huge motivator for any individual to try out new things and follow alternative paths. And I repeat that we unrightfully call them 'alternative'.

Once again, let's get more specific. One of the (as of yet) unbeatable diseases is cancer and its unprecedentedly many life-threatening forms. Chemotherapy was a progress of great value at the beginning of the 20th century. At first, it was not used as a cancer treatment because it was not originally intended as such. So, the era of cancer chemotherapy started out in the 1940s. Since then, cancer treatment development has exploded into a multimillion-dollar industry, of course. Yet, the disease remains the most frequent incurable disease on the planet. Which brings me to my point. When chemotherapy fails – more often than not – people have a tendency to examine all the further choices they have. Giving up is the hardest thing to do – exactly because life is the most precious thing to lose. So, one of the 'alternate' yet logical options that are still left is turn to herbal medicine, for example. And the thought that accompanies it is "It doesn't hurt trying, right?" No, it certainly does not.

At the same time, – this might sound like an oxymoron, but it really isn't – looking back in time can make you appreciate even more every new option, every new "luxurious" item that is available today; especially when talking about medicine and medical progress. In other words, the past is there to give you comfort and to complement modern-day progress. The past is like the grandparent who will always be there to give you the candy that you desire and that no one else will give you – certainly not your parents!

After all, **medicine lives forever,** just like every other science and form of art. Art. Remember when we discussed about medicine being considered a form of art in the past? Well, the debate over the status of medicine as an art or a science is far from resolved. Of course, by art in this case is meant the Aristotelian notion of *techne*, which consists of listening skills directed to the lived experience of the patient in a way that scientific knowledge can be applied therapeutically. The ability to listen to patients is obviously central to the clinician's work and the contention is that it is a skill or art that can be learned. The ancient Greek notion of *techne* is presupposed in clinical practice.

The father of Western medicine, Hippocrates, said **"*Ars longa*"** in one of his aphorisms. Art is long while life is short. People may come and go, but their knowledge and contribution is something that remains. The art of medicine is prior to and independent of medical science which has an important but subordinate role. Medical treatments and diagnostic methods employ highly sophisticated science. But that does not mean that medicine is just applied science, nor that the art of medicine is subordinate to science. Each medical practitioner can acquire lots of skills through study, observation, training, and professional practice. However, if they do not communicate any of their new conclusions and discoveries, this information will disappear along with their demise and that would be a real pity.

As it is a real pity that a big percentage of ancient medical knowledge has been destroyed due to either natural (e.g., corrosion) or anthropogenic (e.g., fire) reasons. Which brings me to the next point I am trying to make, not just with this particular book, but with every book I have published and every other book I may publish in the future. Knowledge and **information is to be spread around**; not to be collecting dust locked away.

Now, let's get back to the debate over whether medicine is **science or art.** At the Renaissance era, Paracelsus (1493-1541) insisted that medicine is a science and an art at the same time. This is an opinion that has seen no disagreement whatsoever. Historically, medicine has not been assigned to one particular category. Now, medicine has surely enlarged basic scientific understanding in numerous fields, such as physiology, nosology, pathology, biochemistry, and so on. In *Cecil Textbook of Medicine*, Lloyd H Smith Jr writes: 'In the art of medicine, the physician must be the advocate of the patient as well as the adversary of disease'. An important step to fully recognizing the significance of medicine alone was the beginning of medical education. Medicine gathered the momentum it has today only by the late 20th century. This ambiguity of being an art and a science has always been there. Medicine is only as "scientific" as the last used cure, but physicians have always pronounced cures, even when they were nothing but the healing powers of nature.

Furthermore, just like every other form of art — apart from living forever — medicine is **ever-evolving.** A disease is now a condition for which medical science provides a cure, and not the other way around. Biomedical discovery is the one that defines the range of clinical problems that a doctor is called to treat. So, we see that even the goals of medicine evolve as time passes. In the Hippocratic era, the basic goal was to cure disease in individual patients. Now, this has — gradually, of course — evolved to a more general goal: eradicate human suffering in the aggregate. This agrees with the new trend in the medical sector: the holistic approach of things.

Another important part of human health that is now a given is **nutrition**. In this time and age, everybody knows that a good and balanced diet combined with proper sleep, rest and regular physical exercise is the best choice for a healthy life — even though only the minority does follow that kind of life. Poor nutrition (which means that nutrition is either improper and too unhealthy or inadequate) can lead to a weakened immune system, and therefore an increased susceptibility to disease, an impaired mental and physical development, and even to reduced productivity. Histories of dietary habits in various national contexts have long been available. In our study, we found out that nutrition's part in health needed to walk a long road to be sufficiently recognized. While famine and pestilence have been associated with human health, it is still unclear enough how and at what point malnutrition starts to compromise one's immunological response.

My advice would be for you to concentrate on the positive effects of a good **diet** and on the benefits each type of food can give you. Psychology is equally important, and rarely does accentuating the negative have the desired results. I mean, concentrating only on strict food policy guidelines about what foods should be eliminated from or limited within our diet because of their fat, sugar, calorie or sodium content seems way too tiring — and for no reason. In the past, people focused on which foods to avoid, what to cut out of their daily diet. Since we have the privilege to live in this time and age, we should not make the same mistakes, especially when it comes to the matter of our health. Please note that the very beginning of medicine as a fully organized activity was when it was indicated that those who were sick required a different diet from those who were well. In the

Scientific Revolution of the 16th and 17th centuries, new ideas emerged concerning the processes of food assimilation, excretion and breathing. Arabic alchemists of previous centuries had placed emphasis upon the principles of liquidity (mercury), metallicity (sulfur), and solidity (salt) in the understanding of chemical reactions. So, by the 16th century, distillation was an established method for extracting the essence from plants and mineral substances.

Today, medicine has reached new highs in almost every way possible and its progress is ongoing. However, we all know that **problems never cease to exist** and modern-day medicine must solve medical-care availability, quantity, quality and distribution issues. To do that, medical research must focus on socioeconomic, political and cultural factors that affect the access to all kinds of medical care and its delivery to the individuals of a community. Such an undertaking must include modern-day domestic-healing networks and also traditional medicine knowledge, especially in Third World countries where resources are very limited. Once again, we find proof that ancient medical knowledge remains useful even to this day. Linking up those social factors with the biological ones and adding an individual's psychology to the mix, we get yet again to the holistic approach of a humanistic medicine.

You may have noticed that I have used the term "holistic medicine" a number of times. To be clearer on the subject, I should add that the holistic healing philosophy of Ancient Greek medicine states that Man is essentially a part and a product of Nature, that is, our natural environment. According to the holistic view of medicine, health is living in harmony with Nature, and disease occurs when this harmony, this balance is disturbed. Thus, healing is the restoration of the lost harmony.

Moving on, I would like to draw your attention to a few more facts. Just like humans, all other living beings on this planet have grown and evolved within the same biosphere. The use of plants for food and of medicinal plants for healing is not exclusive to the human species; an animal that otherwise would be running around free in the wild stops to munch on some healing herbs when it gets sick. It will then get some rest until it feels better. Besides, achieving **wellness through herbal**

medicine first appeared as an imitation of this global healing practice of the animal kingdom. Any system of herbal medicine must have both a theoretical and a practical aspect in order to be sustainable. The theoretical part is necessary to guide the observations and hypotheses of physicians into formulating a diagnostic and treating plan. On the other hand, practical experience is necessary to choose the right herbs and remedies that will be the most effective.

Apart from herbal medicine, another significant feature that we encountered in all five traditional medicines that we studied was a theory that had to do with **nature's elements**. We also saw that all those theories (The Four Humors, The Four Elements, The Five Elements etc.) are closely related. But how did they all come about? It was the early observation that many living creatures were warm while alive and became cold when they died. That was used in explaining the nature of living organisms and the constitution of life itself and it also worked as those theories' initial trigger.

Hippocrates's Four Humors did not correspond just with the four elements of nature but also with temperatures: Blood is warm and moist, phlegm is cold and moist, black bile is cold and dry, and yellow bile is warm and dry. So, we find all four combinations of these two physical properties in our body. Humoral therapy was a mixed one and included diet, exercise, massage, and other modalities that were aimed at the individual needs of the individual patient. The Hippocratics were also acutely aware that diseases often sweep through a community, affecting everybody: the old and young, rich and poor, thin and corpulent, male and female. It was this holistic individualism that was the core feature of their medical practice and, as I said, concerned everybody, irrespectively of social categories. By now, we have established that the fine balance between the four humors, and the four elements as well, accounted for the disposition of an individual towards health or disease.

When **Hippocrates** said, 'Let thy food be thy medicine and thy medicine be thy food,' it was an empirical yet pretty accurate rule. He observed that the more corpulent are more apt to die quickly than the thin and that people who followed a fresh, **plant-based diet** developed fewer diseases. So, he incorporated an improvement of his patients' diet into his treatments. At the time, no one could possibly imagine that in the beginning of the 3rd millennium AD we would be traveling that far back in time to study and use again those words, those wise words that are both our past and our future. Today, we have found out that the link between diet and health has to do with our epigenetics, the study of how lifestyle and environment influence the expression of our genes. The nutrients we extract from food enter metabolic pathways where they are manipulated, modified, and molded into molecules our body can use. One of these pathways is responsible for making methyl groups, that is, important epigenetic tags that suppress genes. Processed foods containing sugar, animal saturated fats and trans fats and artificial chemicals can activate disease-causing genes that might have stayed dormant otherwise.

The Hippocratics strove to take into account several factors when making a diagnosis and recommending a therapeutic regimen. These wider aspects of health and disease were described in the influential treatises '*On Epidemics*' and '*On Airs, Waters, Places*'. The latter is essentially the foundation statement of Western environmentalism, especially as it relates to health and disease. It offered advice on where to build one's house (somewhere where the soil is well-drained and where it is protected from chilling winds), and analyzed the health of communities in terms of the **environmental factors** that affected their inhabitants. The Hippocratics believed that environmental factors could change the basic characteristics of human beings, such as the skin color and the body shape, and that these changes could be passed on to offspring. This is an optimistic philosophy of human malleability, consonant with the general Hippocratic confidence that their therapeutic regimen had much to offer to its patients.

Hippocrates says that to understand the diseases of an area, you have to know what the seasons, winds (weather), and water in the area are like. He connects the study of meteorology and astronomy to the study of medicine. According to Hippocrates, in a place with hot southern winds and salty waters, the people are more overweight, women are sickly and prone to miscarriage, and fevers are typical. In a place with cold winds and waters, the men are thin and wiry and the women have difficult childbirths but don't miscarry often. In places with a moderate climate, with soft waters, there are only a few mild diseases that affect both men and women. Hippocrates went on to describe different types of waters, labeling them as wholesome or unwholesome for drinking depending on their source and the weather of the area around them. He clearly focused on how to predict ailments depending on the seasons, stars, and wind.

Medicine is both a broad science and a personal art at the same time. Its evolution began from the magical invocations of the primitive man towards some higher force. Through a constant observation of the various functions of the body and the mind, people's awe at disease evolved to a systematic scientific methodology aimed to restore the balance between an individual's internal and external environment. Just like with most scientific directions, the foundations of modern medical thought were established in ancient times, within the restless spirit of the Ancient Greek thought. Of course, integrated therapeutic systems were developed not only in Greece, but within the framework of other great civilizations of the past, like those of India and China. After all, it is a known fact that ideas and practices in the past traveled much more than we tend to believe today. In any case, the Ancient Greek thought was the one to constitute the very basis and main point of reference for the long-standing evolution of Western science that has now spread globally.

Greek medicine left three basic principles that formed medicine until the modern period. The **first** principle, as we have already seen, is humoralism. The **second** is the botanical basis of most drugs. Doctors looked to the botanical kingdom for medicines to combat disease. One doctor in particular organized the ancient pharmacopoeia into a form that was proven useful for centuries. Dioscorides wrote a treatise on *Materia Medica* which included the medical-botanical writings of earlier authors and also much of what he himself had discovered about plants and their medicinal qualities. Many botanical preparations, such as opium and hellebore, had great staying power, but unlike the core theoretical content of ancient medicine, plants have definite geographical distributions, and the search for them meant that later doctors had to do their own hunting, in their local forests and hedgerows. Galen incorporated much of Dioscorides' work in his own voluminous writings. The latter's *Materia Medica* was still prized in the Renaissance. The **third** legacy is a secular approach to disease. Both religion and magic continued to influence thinking about health and disease by physicians and laymen. The ancient healers whose writings survived and were prized believed that disease could be understood in natural terms. When Galen or Hippocrates was confronted with a sick patient, they drew on their own knowledge and skills in an attempt to bring about an act of healing.

I remember that, as a schoolkid, the discipline of history was not my cup of tea and when they asked me why, I used to answer that it was lies about periods we have not lived, so it was impossible to know what was going on back then. As I grow older, I can recognize the value and the validity of a historical discovery. Plus, I came to find out that historians think like I used to think as a kid. In fact, for several centuries, medical historians have been interested in the history of... the history of medicine. The study of history itself is not more isolated than any social venture from the critical biological and cultural aspects of disease.

Unfortunately, today, we have a tendency to erase from our memory the study and teachings of the past, the formidable volume of knowledge that was obtained over the centuries, upon which every modern scientific piece of knowledge is based. There would be no civilization, no cultural continuity through time, if it wasn't for the ancient thinkers and intellectuals who put all those questions on the table and searched hard to find answers. Our reconciliation with the perpetual flow of repeated **time** cycles will allow the human thought to create things that stand the test of time and surpass our natural perishability.

The cycles of our historical and scientific course often make us face the same old questions that Ionian philosophers faced; the very nature of still-unsolved health problems makes it almost imperative for us to study the past and use it as a source of wisdom for the future. The abundance, the richness of theoretical thought and practical application that bloomed in the medical field of Ancient Greece is of paramount importance on a global scale and is also something worth revisiting over and over in our scientific and moral course.

The history of medicine in recent decades has opened a new window on the past, increasing the need for a distinction between medical history and social history. Calling into question the traditional functionalist notions of medicine has spawned the new social history of medicine, about which I will write in another book. There are social issues of crucial importance such as gender and sexuality, race, social class, and ethnicity, that should be further investigated as they related to health, disease, and medicine in the past.

Periodically, the already existing historical literature has been the subject of meticulous review in order for it to be properly and as accurately as possible validated and verified. Even for medical history, there are many directions through which we can study and analyze it. The study of the history of medicine will necessarily continue to change in the future as medicine and its meaning, nature and knowledge base continue to change. The present will continue to shape our questions, approaches, and concerns. In the years ahead, historians of medicine will look again to the past and will search for new and more sophisticated ways of understanding the present and facing the future.

APPENDIX 1

The Hippocratic Oath in Ancient Greek

Ὄμνυμι Ἀπόλλωνα ἰητρὸν, καὶ Ἀσκληπιὸν, καὶ Ὑγείαν, καὶ Πανάκειαν, καὶ θεούς πάντας τε καὶ πάσας, ἵστορας ποιεύμενος, ἐπιτελέα ποιήσειν κατὰ δύναμιν καὶ κρίσιν ἐμὴν ὅρκον τόνδε καὶ ξυγγραφὴν τήνδε.

Ἡγήσασθαι μὲν τὸν διδάξαντά με τὴν τέχνην ταύτην ἴσα γενέτῃσιν ἐμοῖσι, καὶ βίου κοινώσασθαι, καὶ χρεῶν χρηίζοντι μετάδοσιν ποιήσασθαι, καὶ γένος τὸ ἐξ ωὐτέου ἀδελφοῖς ἴσον ἐπικρινέειν ἄρρεσι, καὶ διδάξειν τὴν τέχνην ταύτην, ἢν χρηίζωσι μανθάνειν, ἄνευ μισθοῦ καὶ ξυγγραφῆς, παραγγελίης τε καὶ ἀκροήσιος καὶ τῆς λοιπῆς ἁπάσης μαθήσιος μετάδοσιν ποιήσασθαι υἱοῖσί τε ἐμοῖσι, καὶ τοῖσι τοῦ ἐμὲ διδάξαντος, καὶ μαθηταῖσι συγγεγραμμένοισί τε καὶ ὠρκισμένοις νόμῳ ἰητρικῷ, ἄλλῳ δὲ οὐδενί.

Διαιτήμασί τε χρήσομαι ἐπ' ὠφελείῃ καμνόντων κατὰ δύναμιν καὶ κρίσιν ἐμήν, ἐπὶ δηλήσει δὲ καὶ ἀδικίῃ εἴρξειν.

Οὐ δώσω δὲ οὐδὲ φάρμακον οὐδενὶ αἰτηθεὶς θανάσιμον, οὐδὲ ὑφηγήσομαι ξυμβουλίην τοιήνδε. Ὁμοίως δὲ οὐδὲ γυναικὶ πεσσὸν φθόριον δώσω. Ἁγνῶς δὲ καὶ ὁσίως διατηρήσω βίον τὸν ἐμὸν καὶ τέχνην τὴν ἐμήν.

Οὐ τεμέω δὲ οὐδὲ μὴν λιθιῶντας, ἐκχωρήσω δὲ ἐργάτῃσιν ἀνδράσι πρήξιος τῆσδε.

Ἐς οἰκίας δὲ ὁκόσας ἂν ἐσίω, ἐσελεύσομαι ἐπ' ὠφελείῃ καμνόντων, ἐκτὸς ἐὼν πάσης ἀδικίης ἑκουσίης καὶ φθορίης, τῆς τε ἄλλης καὶ ἀφροδισίων ἔργων ἐπί τε γυναικείων σωμάτων καὶ ἀνδρῴων, ἐλευθέρων τε καὶ δούλων.

Ἃ δ' ἂν ἐν θεραπείῃ ἢ ἴδω, ἢ ἀκούσω, ἢ καὶ ἄνευ θεραπηίης κατὰ βίον ἀνθρώπων, ἃ μὴ χρή ποτε ἐκλαλέεσθαι ἔξω, σιγήσομαι, ἄρρητα ἡγεύμενος εἶναι τὰ τοιαῦτα.

Ὅρκον μὲν οὖν μοι τόνδε ἐπιτελέα ποιέοντι, καὶ μὴ ξυγχέοντι, εἴη ἐπαύρασθαι καὶ βίου καὶ τέχνης δοξαζομένῳ παρὰ πᾶσιν ἀνθρώποις ἐς τὸν αἰεὶ χρόνον. παραβαίνοντι δὲ καὶ ἐπιορκοῦντι, τἀναντία τουτέων.

APPENDIX 2

The Hippocratic Oath in Modern English

I swear to fulfill, to the best of my ability and judgment, this covenant: ...

I will respect the hard-won scientific gains of those physicians in whose steps I walk, and gladly share such knowledge as is mine with those who are to follow.

I will apply, for the benefit of the sick, all measures which are required, avoiding those twin traps of overtreatment and therapeutic nihilism.

I will remember that there is art to medicine as well as science, and that warmth, sympathy, and understanding may outweigh the surgeon's knife or the chemist's drug.

I will not be ashamed to say, "I know not," nor will I fail to call in my colleagues when the skills of another are needed for a patient's recovery.

I will respect the privacy of my patients, for their problems are not disclosed to me that the world may know. Most especially must I tread with care in matters of life and death. Above all, I must not play at God.

I will remember that I do not treat a fever chart, a cancerous growth, but a sick human being, whose illness may affect the person's family and economic stability. My responsibility includes these related problems, if I am to care adequately for the sick.

I will prevent disease whenever I can, for prevention is preferable to cure.

I will remember that I remain a member of society, with special obligations to all my fellow human beings, those sound of mind and body as well as the infirm.

If I do not violate this oath, may I enjoy life and art, respected while I live and remembered with affection thereafter. May I always act so as to preserve the finest traditions of my calling and may I long experience the joy of healing those who seek my help.

Written in 1964 by Louis Lasagna, Academic Dean of the School of Medicine at Tufts University.

APPENDIX 3

The following table is but a limited summary of the best part of my study. Cataloguing the entire list of medicinal herbs and plants and every little ailment (such as headaches and fever) that each one treats or helps treat would result in an unmanageably long and not easy-to-use table. So, only the basic types of health problems are here together with at least one of the herbs that were (thought to be) effective for their cure.

Condition\Country	China	Egypt	Greece	India	Iran
Cardiovascular problems	Motherwort	Onion	Olive	Arjuna	Agarwood, Haoma
Diarrhea	Blackberry, Raspberry	Acacia	Witch-hazel	Ashoka	Skullcap, Squaw vine
Eye diseases	Wolfberry, Chrysanthemum, Rehmannia	Castor oil	Clary sage	Amla, Harad	Hollyhock, Jujube
Infections	Coptis	Honey	Houseleek, Snapdragon	Rakta chitrak	Garlic & Rue
Pain relief	Alangium	Coriander	Nicotiana, Opium poppy	Ashoka, Rakta chitrak	Bangha
Respiratory disorders	Liquorice	Hibiscus	Yarrow	Guggul	Frankincense, Haoma
Sexual disorders	Dong quai	Fenugreek	Parsley	Curry, Drumsticks	Pomegranate

Skin diseases	Wolfberry	Henna	Evening primrose, Valerian	Garlic (ajoene)	Calendula (marigold)
Stomach disorders	Cardamom	Caraway	Mint, Saffron	Hogweed	Assyrian plum
Vitality	Ginseng	Garlic	Fennel	Guggul	Sandalwood

SOURCES

https://draxe.com/two-ancient-superfoods-join-forces/?utm_source=newsletter&utm_medium=email&utm_campaign=bbpt-advertorial

http://www.scienceinschool.org/2014/issue28/epigenetics

http://advances.nutrition.org/content/1/1/8.full

http://www.epigenome.eu/en/2,48,872

http://www.epigenome.eu/en/1,38,0

https://www.functionalmedicine.org/What_is_Functional_Medicine/AboutFM/

https://draxe.com/traditional-chinese-medicine/

http://kaleidoscope.cultural-china.com/en/118Kaleidoscope3138.html

http://tvxs.gr/news/ygeia/mnimi-i-giogka-einai-kalyteri-apo-ta-stayroleksa

http://www.huffingtonpost.gr/2016/05/15/egoimhsh_n_9978896.html?utm_hp_ref=greece

http://www.huffingtonpost.gr/2014/11/19/ippokratis-omoiopathitiki-7-therapeftika-votana_n_6151440.html

http://www.acupuncturetoday.com/mpacms/at/article.php?id=28498

http://www.nytimes.com/2016/09/24/world/asia/chinese-medicine-paul-unschuld.html?_r=0

http://jpkc.shutcm.edu.cn/yxyy/part06/teaching-cases/2010%20%E4%B8%AD%E5%8C%BB%E8%8B%B1%E8%AF%AD%E7%9F%A5%E8%AF%86%E7%AB%9E%E8%B5%9B/%E6%B8%A9%E7%8F%AE%E5%BD%A4-QI%20BO%20AND%20HIPPOCRATES.pdf

http://www.schizas.com/site3/index.php?option=com_content&view=article&id=43925%3A2011-04-19-170000&catid=50%3Amathaino-tin-ellada&Itemid=336&lang=el

http://www.schizas.com/site3/index.php?option=com_content&view=article&id=2195%3A2009-11-21-16-58-50&catid=50%3Amathaino-tin-ellada&Itemid=336&lang=el#ixzz4DBGwdWoO

http://www.schizas.com/site3/index.php?option=com_content&view=article&id=4039%3A2010-05-31-18-59-43&catid=24%3Akatxriseis-i-xrrisima&Itemid=203&lang=el#ixzz4DBdxbYUH

http://www.protothema.gr/world/article/620181/arhaia-adikatathliptika-vrethikan-se-arhaioelliniki-poli-stin-tourkia/

http://www.sciencemag.org/sites/default/files/custom-publishing/documents/TCM_Dec_19_issue_high_resolution.pdf

http://www.sciencemag.org/sites/default/files/custom-publishing/documents/TCM_Jan_16_2015_high%20res.pdf

http://www.sciencemag.org/sites/default/files/custom-publishing/documents/TCM3_Nov%2013_issue2.pdf

http://eranistis.net/wordpress/2013/03/27/%CE%BF-%CE%B9%CF%80%CF%80%CE%BF%CE%BA%CF%81%CE%AC%CF%84%CE%B7%CF%82-%CE%BA%CE%B1%CE%B9-%CE%B7-%CE%B9%CE%B1%CF%84%CF%81%CE%B9%CE%BA%CE%AE-

%CF%84%CF%89%CE%BD-%CE%B1%CF%81%CF%87%CE%B1%CE%AF%CF%89%CE%BD/

http://www.schizas.com/site3/index.php?option=com_content&view=article&id=2195:2009-11-21-16-58-50&catid=50:mathaino-tin-ellada&Itemid=336

http://www.skai.gr/news/technology/article/159195/to-meli-apotelei-adidoto-sta-eortastika-methusia-/

http://www.solon.org.gr/index.php/epistimes-anthropou/111-2008-07-15-18-39-07/1476-glossa-tis-therapeias.html

http://aromafarm.gr/article-categories/268-%CF%84%CE%B1-%CE%B2%CF%8C%CF%84%CE%B1%CE%BD%CE%B1-%CF%83%CF%84%CE%B7%CE%BD-%CE%B1%CF%81%CF%87%CE%B1%CE%AF%CE%B1-%CE%B1%CE%B9%CE%B3%CF%85%CF%80%CF%84%CE%B9%CE%B1%CE%BA%CE%AE-%CE%B9%CE%B1%CF%84%CF%81%CE%B9%CE%BA%CE%AE

https://explorable.com/islamic-medicine

http://www.sciencemuseum.org.uk/broughttolife

http://www.muslimphilosophy.com/ip/rep/H018.htm

http://www.muslimphilosophy.com/ip/rep/H010.htm

http://www.muslimphilosophy.com/ip/rep/H001.htm

http://www.muslimphilosophy.com/ip/rep/H002

http://www.muslimphilosophy.com/ip/rep/H011

https://www.oc.edu/dotAsset/af7c1211-793c-499c-8e00-b243f6a50494.pdf

http://www.islamicmedicine.org/alrazi3.htm

http://www.muslimheritage.com/uploads/
The Valuable Contributions of al-Razi in the History of Pharmacy.pdf

http://www.muslimphilosophy.com/ip/rep/H043.htm

https://www.omorfizoi.gr/sygkritikh-meleth-arxaias-ellhnikhs-kai-kinezikhs-iatrikhs/

http://spiros-reflexologia.blogspot.gr/2008/10/blog-post.html

http://www.nytimes.com/2016/09/24/world/asia/chinese-medicine-paul-unschuld.html?_r=0

http://cn.nytimes.com/china/20151014/c14sino-paul-qa/en-us/

http://www.akadimia.gr/%CF%83%CF%85%CE%BD%CE%AD%CE%BD%CF%84%CE%B5%CF%85%CE%BE%CE%B7-%CF%84%CE%BF%CF%85-paul-unschuld-%CE%BC%CE%B5-%CF%84%CE%BF%CE%BD-%CE%B1%CE%BB%CE%AD%CE%BE%CE%B1%CE%BD%CE%B4%CF%81%CE%BF-%CF%84%CE%B7%CE%BB/

http://www.independent.co.uk/arts-entertainment/books/reviews/blood-guts-a-short-history-of-medicine-by-roy-porter-134878.html

https://dash.harvard.edu/bitstream/handle/1/3372913/Brandt_Emerging.pdf?sequence=1

http://mh.bmj.com/content/28/2/74.full

http://flowingzen.com/15937/the-15-most-frequently-asked-questions-about-qigong/

http://jprsolutions.info/files/final-file-57216ece615432.92287015.pdf

http://iranian.com/main/blog/m-saadat-noury/happy-razi-day-first-iranian-famous-chemist-mohammad-zakariya-razi.html

BOOKS

Barritt, P., 2005. *Humanity in healthcare: the heart and soul of medicine.* Radcliffe Publishing.

Bhatia, S.L., 1972. *Medical science in ancient India.* Department of Publications and Extension Lectures, Bangalore University.

Bhishagratna, K.L. ed., 1907. *An English translation of the Sushruta Samhita based on original Sanskrit text (Vol. 1).* Wilkin's Press.

Browne, E.G., 2001. *Islamic medicine: Fitzpatrick lectures delivered at the Royal College of Physicians in 1919-1920.* Goodword Books.

Bunn M., 2010. *Ancient Wisdom for Modern Health: Rediscover the Simple, Timeless Secrets of Health and Happiness.* Enlightened Health Publishing.

Bynum, W.F. and Porter, R., 2013. *Companion encyclopedia of the history of medicine.* Routledge.

Christie, D., 2013. *Thirty Years in Moukden, 1883-1913.* Theclassics Us.

Cullen, C. and Lo, V., 2004. *Medieval Chinese medicine: the Dunhuang medical manuscripts.* Routledge.

Efthymiou-Egleton, I., 2016. *Do We Really Know China? An Outsider's View.* XLIBRIS.

Efthymiou-Egleton, I., 2016. *Trends in Health Care: A Global Challenge.* XLIBRIS

Frye, R.N., 2000. *The golden age of Persia: the Arabs in the East.* Sterling Publishing Company.

Gignoux, P., 2001. *Man and cosmos in ancient Iran.* Istituto italiano per l'Africa e l'Oriente.

Gordon, R., 1997. *The alarming history of medicine: Amusing anecdotes from Hippocrates to heart transplants.* Macmillan.

Grof, S. and Valier, M.L. eds., 1984. *Ancient wisdom and modern science.* SUNY Press.

Hoeber, P.B., 1935. Annals of Medical History. *British medical journal,* 2(3887), p.41.

Jackson, M., 2011. *The Oxford handbook of the history of medicine.* Oxford University Press on Demand.

Jaggi, O.P., 1984. *History of Science, Technology and Medicine in India: Technology in Modern India.* Atma Ram and Sons.

Keswani, N.H. ed., 1974. *The Science of Medicine and Physiological Concepts in Ancient & Medieval India.* All-India Institute of Medical Sciences.

Meulenbeld, G.J., 2000. *A history of Indian medical literature* (Vol. 2). Groningen.

Mitchell, W.E., 1977. Changing others: the anthropological study of therapeutic systems. *Medical Anthropology Newsletter,* 8(3), pp.15-20.

Mijares, S.G., 2014. *Modern psychology and ancient wisdom: Psychological healing practices from the world's religious traditions.* Routledge.

Moss, C.A., 2010. *Power of the five elements: the Chinese medicine path to healthy aging and stress resistance.* North Atlantic Books.

O'Malley, C.D. ed., 1970. *The History of medical education: an international symposium held February 5-9, 1968* (Vol. 12). Univ of California Press.

Pregadio, F., 2006. *Great clarity: Daoism and alchemy in early medieval China.* Stanford University Press.

Porter, R., 2001. *The Cambridge illustrated history of medicine.* Cambridge University Press.

Prioreschi, P., 2003. *A history of medicine: Roman medicine* (Vol. 3). Edwin Mellen Press.

Redfern, G., 2009. *Ancient Wisdoms: Exploring the Mysteries and Connections.* AuthorHouse.

Risse, G.B., 1991. The history of therapeutics. *Essays in the History of Therapeutics*, pp.3-11.

Roth R. and Occhiogrosso P., 2001. *Holy Spirit for Healing: Merging Ancient Wisdom with Modern Medicine.* Hay House

Schayegh, C., 1900. Who is Knowledgeable is Strong: Science. *Class, and the Formation of Modern Iranian Society, 1950*, pp.95-103.

Sigerist, H.E., 1987. *A history of medicine: Early Greek, Hindu, and Persian medicine* (No. 27). New York: Oxford University Press.

Sigerist, H.E., 1952. A History of Medicine. Vol. I. Primitive and Archaic Medicine.

Strathern, P., 2005. *A brief history of medicine: from Hippocrates to gene therapy.* Running Press.

Thaker, P.B., 1995. Philosophical foundations in ancient Indian medicine: Science, philosophy, and ethics in" Caraka-samhita".

Tucker, E., 2016. *The Middle East in Modern World History.* Routledge.

Vogel, M.J. and Rosenberg, C.E., 1979. The therapeutic revolution: Essays in the social history of American medicine.

Yar-Shater, E., 2004. *The history of Medicine in Iran.* Bibliotheca Persica.

Zysk, K.G., 1992. *Religious Medicine: The History and Evolution of Indian Medicine.* Transaction Publishers.

Zysk, K.G., 1998. *Asceticism and healing in ancient India: medicine in the Buddhist monastery* (Vol. 2). Motilal Banarsidass Publishe.

Guenter B. Risse. The History of Therapeutics, Clio Medica, 1991; 22:3-11.

The historical relations of ancient Hindu with Greek medicine in connection with the study of Modern Medical Science in India. A general introductory lecture delivered June 1850 at Calcutta Medical College. By Allan Webb, J.C. Sherriff, Military Orphan Press 1850

Suśruta saṁhitā: text with English translation, a full and comprehensive introduction, additional text, different readings, notes, comparative views, index, glossary and plates, Volume 3
Suśruta, Kunjalal Bhishagratna
Chowkhamba Sanskrit Series Office, Feb 1, 1999

Philosophical Foundations in Ancient Indian Medicine: Science, Philosophy, and Ethics in Caraka-Samhita
Pramod B. Thaker, Boston College, 1995

MD: Medical Newsmagazine, Volume 9
MD Publications, 1965

Medical Anthropology: Traditional Medicine, Robert A. Rubinstein, the Spirit Catches You and You Fall Down, Ethnomedicine
Books, LLC, 2010

Annals of Medical History
Francis Randolph Packard
P.B. Hoeber., 1930

Ancient Wisdom: Modern World Paperback – January 6, 2000
by Dalai Lama XIV Bstan-'dzin-rgya-mtsho

The Alarming History of Medicine: Amusing Anecdotes from Hippocrates to Heart Transplants
Richard Gordon, St. Martin's Press, Sep 15, 1997

Ancient Wisdom and Modern Science
edited by Stanislav Grof, Marjorie Livingston Valier
State University of New York Press, 1984

A History of Medicine: Greek medicine
By Plinio Prioreschi, 1993

www.ingramcontent.com/pod-product-compliance
Lightning Source LLC
Chambersburg PA
CBHW030931180526
45163CB00002B/526